A Guide to
School Services in
Speech-Language Pathology

TRICI SCHRAEDER, MS, CCC-SLP

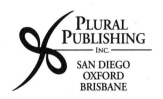

PLURAL
PUBLISHING
INC.

SAN DIEGO
OXFORD
BRISBANE

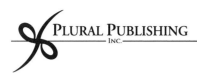

5521 Ruffin Road
San Diego, CA 92123

e-mail: info@pluralpublishing.com
Web site: http://www.pluralpublishing.com

49 Bath Street
Abingdon, Oxfordshire OX14 1EA
United Kingdom

Typeset in 11/13 Garamond by Flanagan's Publishing Services, Inc.
Printed in the United States of America by McNaughton and Gunn

Library of Congress Cataloging in Publication Data

Schraeder, Trici.
  A guide to school services in speech-language pathology / Trici Schraeder.
     p. ; cm.
  Includes bibliographical references and index.
  ISBN-13: 978-1-59756-179-2 (pbk.)
  ISBN-10: 1-59756-179-7 (pbk.)
  1. Speech therapy for children—United States. I. Title.
  [DNLM: 1. Speech-Language Pathology—United States. 2. School Health Services—United States.
WL 340.2 S377s 2007]
  LB3454.S368 2007
    371.91'42—dc22
                                                   2006103403

Contents

Preface

A Guide to School Services in Speech-Language Pathology is about the exciting world of the school-based speech-language pathologist and current issues related to providing speech-language services in public schools. As illustrated throughout the book by numerous examples of challenging professional scenarios, interesting clinical interventions, and successful applications, the school setting can be a complex and highly stimulating practice venue.

This book is presented as an introductory overview for the college student who is ready to embark on his or her school-based student teaching experience. Although it is tailored to the needs of the novice practitioner, many of the experienced professionals who served as peer reviewers commented that the book also would be a useful resource for the professional, school-based speech-language pathologist.

The book is organized to take the reader on a quick walk through American history related to school-based speech-language pathology services and then lead the reader to information about modern-day issues. In this way the reader may acquire an appreciation for the social, political, cultural, demographic, economic, and research-based influences that have shaped how school-based speech-language pathology services have evolved, and continue to evolve, over time. Current legal mandates are discussed (e.g., the Individuals with Disabilities Education Improvement Act, the No Child Left Behind Act, the Americans with Disabilities Act). The preferred practice patterns of the speech-language pathologist, as defined by the American Speech-Language-Hearing Association (ASHA), are intertwined into the content of every chapter, along with many of the guidelines and position statements set forth by the ASHA. The

lists of references presented at the end of each chapter serve to confirm that all of the information presented relates to evidence-based practice and provide the advanced learner with a means to explore topics in greater depth.

The reader is introduced to the necessary knowledge base, skills, and dispositions of the professional speech-language pathologist. Cutting-edge service delivery models are described. The concept of a workload analysis approach to establishing caseload standards in schools is introduced, and implementation strategies are offered. Concrete, real-life success stories are shared. Strategies for using evidence-based practice, proactive behavior management, conflict resolution, professional collaboration, conferencing and counseling skills, cultural competencies, goal writing, informal assessment procedures, and creating testing accommodations are offered. Real-life scenarios based on experiences shared by public school speech-language pathologists give the reader concrete examples on which to scaffold the complex professional concepts. Chapter summaries provide an overview of major points related to the material presented. Questions at the end of each chapter are designed to engage the reader in cognitive exercises at the analysis, application, synthesis, and evaluation levels of thinking as well as the knowledge and comprehension levels of thinking. Relevant vocabulary terms are defined at the start of each chapter. These terms were identified by a University of Wisconsin–Madison undergraduate student who had taken an introductory course in the field. That student highlighted the vocabulary words that were unknown to him while reading a draft of the book for the first time. Thus, the perspective of the new learner has been taken into consideration.

Acknowledgments

It is with deep appreciation that I acknowledge the contribution of Linda R. Schreiber, MS, CCC-SLP, Consultant and Board-Recognized Specialist in Child Language. Without Linda's editorial consultation services, this book would not have been published.

The colleagues named in the following list served as peer reviewers. Their professional insights are highly valued, and their dedication to the field is unsurpassed.

Susan Bartlett, MA, CCC-SLP, University of Connecticut, Glastonbury, CT

Patricia Bellini, MA, CCC-SLP, Providence, RI

Jeri Berman, MA, CCC-SLP, ASHA Office, Rockville, MD

Andrea Bertone, MS, CCC-SLP, Madison Area School District, Madison, WI

Larry Biehl, MS, CCC-SLP, Tucson, AZ

Robert Burke, MA, retired fifth grade teacher, Janesville, WI

Nina Cass, MS, CCC-SLP, Amherst, WI

Ingrid Curcio, MS, CCC-SLP, Madison Area School District, Madison, WI

Sally Disney, MS, CCC-SLP, Hamilton County ESC, Loveland, OH

Alyson Eith, MS, CCC-SLP, Madison Area School District, Madison, WI

Kathy Erdman, MS, CCC-SLP, Marquette University, Milwaukee, WI

Susan Floyd, PhD, CCC-SLP, South Carolina Department of Public Instruction, Lake City, SC

Chris Freiberg, MS, CCC-SLP, Wausau Area School District, Wausau, WI

Cindy Forster, MS, CCC-SLP, UW-Stevens Point, Stevens Point, WI

Marycarolyn Jagodzinski, MS, CCC-SLP, CESA #8, Gillett, WI

Mary Anne Jones, MS, CCC-SLP, Las Vegas, NV

Pete Knotek, MS, CCC-SLP, Racine Area School District, Racine, WI

Heidi Notbohm, MS, CCC-SLP, Middleton/Cross Plains Area School District, Middleton, WI

De Anne Wellman-Owre, MS, CCC-SLP, North Smithfield, RI

Barb Rademaker, MA, CCC-SLP, Wausau, WI

Gwen Robl, MS, CCC-SLP, Waunakee Area School District, Waunakee, WI

Judy Rudebusch, EdD, CCC-SLP, Irving, TX

Jeremy Schraeder, BA, Information Technology Specialist, Madison, WI

Sheryl Squier Thormann, MS, CCC-SLP, Speech-Language Program Consultant, Department of Public Instruction, Madison, WI

Jamie Thomas, MS, CCC-SLP, Fort Worth, TX

Kathleen Whitmire, PhD, CCC-SLP, ASHA Office, Rockville, MD

Pat Wildgen, MS, CCC-SLP, Madison Area School District, Madison, WI

Permission to adapt material from the following sources used in Chapter 2 is gratefully acknowledged:

■ American Speech-Language-Hearing Association. (2002). *A workload analysis approach to caseload standards in schools*. Rockville, MD: Author.

- American Speech-Language-Hearing Association. (2003). *Implementation guide: A workload analysis approach to caseload standards in schools.* Rockville, MD: Author.
- Middleton/Cross Plains Area School District. (2005a). *Speech/language severity rating scale: Elementary level.* Unpublished manuscript, Middleton, WI.
- Middleton/Cross Plains Area School District. (2005b). *Speech/language severity rating scale: Secondary level.* Unpublished manuscript, Middleton, WI.

The members of the ASHA Workload/Caseload ad hoc committee were Frank Cirrin and Ann Bird, co-chairs, and, in alphabetical order, Larry Biehl, Sally Disney, Ellen Estomin, Judy Rudebusch, Trici Schraeder, and Kathleen Whitmire (ex officio). Heidi Notbohm served as chairperson of the Middleton/Cross Plains Area School District SLP Workload Weighting System ad hoc committee.

Readers have permission to photocopy the Oral Language Curriculum Standards Inventory (OL-CSI), found on pages 170 to 188, for clinical purposes.

I dedicate this book to my family,
who have blessed me with so many rich and rewarding life experiences
through many years of dynamic, energized, interesting, creative, heart-warming,
challenging, and loving acts of communication.

Chapter 1

ORIGINS OF PUBLIC SCHOOL SPEECH-LANGUAGE PATHOLOGY PROGRAMS

RELATED VOCABULARY

American Speech-Language-Hearing Association (ASHA) The professional association that promotes the interests of speech-language pathologists and audiologists, ensures ethical practices and the highest-quality services, and advocates for persons with communication disorders.

adequate yearly progress (AYP) A provision in the No Child Left Behind Act that requires each state to implement a statewide accountability system that documents how students are making expected academic progress, as defined by academic standards, each school year.

clinical fellowship A program in which, during the first year of professional employment, the novice speech-language pathologist receives mentoring by a professional who holds a Certificate of Clinical Competence (CCC) from the American Speech-Language-Hearing Association. The fellowship supervisor must complete a total of 36 monitoring activities throughout the clinical program, including 18 on-site observations and 18 other monitoring activities, which must be documented. The novice must complete a successful clinical fellowship in order to acquire a CCC.

cognitive-developmental model A service delivery approach in which the speech-language pathologist (SLP) first determines the stage of cognitive development, as described by Jean Piaget, that the child exhibits through overt behaviors. Then the SLP structures the environment and linguistic input to enhance the child's learning processes within that developmental stage.

disaggregated results When a school district reports student scores on statewide assessments for the purposes of documenting adequate yearly progress, the scores of students with disabilities, students who are English language learners, students from low socioeconomic backgrounds, and students from specific ethnic groups must be reported separately. These separated scores are known as disaggregated results.

highest qualified provider A term that currently is defined differently in each state. The American Speech-Language-Hearing Association (ASHA) advocates for the definition to mean a professional who holds an ASHA Certificate of Clinical Competence. Currently, however, many states define the term to mean a person who holds a license in the area of exceptionality.

Individuals with Disabilities Education Improvement Act (IDEA '04) The federal law, reauthorized in 2004, that ensures the right of all children with a disability, 3 to 21 years of age, to receive a free and appropriate public education in the least restrictive environment and also ensures the due process rights of the parents or legal guardians.

individualized education program (IEP) The process and product that ensures that a student with a disability, between the ages of 3 and 21 years, will receive a free and appropriate education in the least restrictive environment. The IEP must be created by a team that includes the parent or legal guardian. The IEP reflects the student's current performance, annual goals, participation with nondisabled peers, participation in statewide and districtwide testing, and, with regard to special education and related services, when those services will begin, how often they will be given, and how long they will last; how progress will be measured; how the parents or legal guardians will be informed of the progress; and the transition services that are needed. The IEP is updated at least every academic year.

individual family service plan (IFSP) The process and product that ensures that a child with a disability, between birth and the age of 3 years, and his or her family receive the services they need to achieve outcomes implemented in a natural environment. The IFSP reflects who will provide the services and where, how often, and how long they will be provided. The IFSP is updated at least every 6 months.

inclusive practices The educational mandate of bringing special education and support services to the student requiring them in the least restrictive environment through a collaborative team effort.

Knowledge and Skills Acquisition (KASA) A document created by the American Speech-Language-Hearing Association (ASHA) that delineates all of the academic and clinical standards set forth by the ASHA that describe what a speech-language pathologist should know and be able to do on completion of a master's degree program.

least restrictive environment (LRE)   The educational mandate that, to the maximum extent possible, a student with a disability should be educated with his or her nondisabled peers. IDEA '04 dictates that the LRE should be the regular education classroom, and that whenever special education and support services need to be provided in a setting other than the regular education classroom, the IEP team must document why it is necessary to provide the services in an alternative setting.

lisp   Misarticulation of the s, z, sh, ch, or j sound due to misplacement of the tongue or abnormalities of articulatory mechanisms.

mainstreaming   A program format that was the precursor to inclusive practices; the student with disabilities was pulled out of the classroom for special education and related services. He or she participated in the regular education classroom for only a small portion of the day, to build social skills.

meta-cognition   Thinking about one's own thinking. Understanding one's own executive functions (e.g., problem-solving, categorization, memorizing) and reflecting on how one accomplishes those functions.

neurogenic speech disorder   A speech impairment that is the result of dysfunction of the neurological system or combined dysfunction of the muscles and nerves.

para-educator   A person who has acquired a 2-year technical degree that prepares him or her to function as an assistant, with a limited scope of practice, under the supervision of a fully certified speech-language pathologist.

pedagogy   The art or the profession of teaching.

speech correctionist   The first term created in 1925 by the American Academy of Speech Correction to describe the professional who practices speech-language pathology.

speech impairment The deterioration, weakening, or partial loss of function which may be the result of an injury, malformation, or disease.

speech impediment An outdated term used as a synonym for speech impairment.

speech-language pathologist (SLP)   A professional trained to provide services for the person who exhibits a communication delay, disorder, or difference resulting from an impairment of articulation, voice, fluency, swallowing, hearing, cognitive aspects of language, social aspects of language, or language comprehension or production, or requires an alternative communication modality.

speech-language pathology   The professional field that focuses on the prevention, etiology, diagnosis, prognosis, and treatment of communication delays, disorders, or differences in the realm of articulation, fluency, voice, resonance, swallowing, cognitive aspects of communication, social aspects of communication, various communication modalities, or the effect of hearing on communication.

stammer, stammering   An outdated term that describes a disorder of speech fluency, rhythm, rate, or involuntary speech stoppage and the emotions the speaker feels before, during, or after the event of fluency disruption.

stutter   A disruption in the fluency, timing, or patterning of speech and the speaker's emotional reaction before, during, or after the event. Primary characteristics may include, but are not limited to, audible or inaudible laryngeal tension, sound, syllable or word repetitions, sound prolongations, interjections, partial word abandonment, and circumlocutions. Secondary characteristics may accompany the primary characteristics. The disturbance may be at the level of neuromuscular, respiratory, laryngeal, or articulatory mechanisms.

Introduction

During the first century of U.S. history, no **speech-language pathology** services were offered in public schools. To understand why this was the case, one must first understand the status of child labor laws in the United States during that era. As early as the 1800s, states and territories enacted more than 1,600 laws protecting children from exploitation in the work force. Nevertheless, it was very common for children in rural areas to toil every waking hour with their parents doing farm work. Hard labor for the sake of the family's survival often took precedence over education. The strong work ethic was also prevalent in urban areas where children and their parents worked in mills, foundries, and factories. Throughout the 1800s, local child labor laws did not apply to immigrant children whose entire families worked for a single company, lived in company-owned homes, and typically worked 68 to 72 hours per week. The U.S. Supreme Court from that era repeatedly yielded to the political pressures applied by factory owners and ruled that child labor laws were unconstitutional. In 1907, Congress chartered the National Child Labor Committee (NCLC) at the persistent request of socially concerned citizens and politicians. As documented by The History Place (1998), the concerns of the NCLC came into national focus when photographs by Lewis Hine publicized the deplorable life experiences of young children in America.

Lewis Hine (1874–1940) was a teacher born in Oshkosh, Wisconsin who gave up his career as an educator to become a photographer for the NCLC. Hine traveled across the United States from 1908 to 1912 documenting and photographing children working long hours in dingy, unsafe conditions. Hine published his first of many photo essays in 1909. Hine's photo essays created national publicity that led to many states banning the employment of underage children. Public education of young children became a national initiative in the early 1900s when droves of children left the farm fields, foundries, mills, and factories and began attending public schools on a regular basis. The incidence of communication disorders among children became known when more children started attending public schools.

Speech correction program was the term used to describe speech-language pathology services in the early 1900s. The first states to develop speech correction programs included Wisconsin, New York, Illinois, Ohio, and Michigan (Neidecker & Blosser, 1993; Taylor, 1992). The first college training program for prospective communication specialists was established at the University of Wisconsin-Madison, and the first doctor of philosophy degree in the United States in the field of speech correction was granted to Sara M. Stinchfield-Hawk at the University of Wisconsin-Madison in 1921. Wisconsin was also the first state to enact enabling legislation for public school speech services. In 1923, Wisconsin appointed a state supervisor of speech correction at the Department of Public Instruction. By 1924, speech correction programs were prevalent in public schools in cities on the east and west coasts of the United States. The American Academy of Speech Correction, now known as the **American Speech-Language-Hearing Association** (ASHA), had 25 professional members in 1926.

The early speech correction programs mirrored a medical model, primarily because physicians were the advocates who shaped the knowledge, skills, and attitudes of those early **speech correctionists**. In the medical model, the professional focused on the problem and cured or diminished its symptoms. One of the pioneers in the field was E. W. Scripture, PhD (Leipzig), MD (Munich). Dr. Scripture had a distinguished career: He was Associate in Psychiatry at Columbia University, Director of the Research Laboratory of Neurology at Vanderbilt Clinic, formerly an assistant professor of experimental psychology at Yale University, and the author of one of the first texts ever written about communication disorders. Although Scripture was an advocate for speech-language services, his attitude toward children who had communication disabilities—specifically, those manifesting as **stutter** and **lisp**—appeared to be somewhat harsh and condescending (1912):

> It would be difficult to find a group of people more neglected by medicine and **pedagogy** than that of stutterers and lispers. The stuttering children that encumber the schools are a source of merriment to their comrades, a torment to themselves, and an irritating distraction to the teacher. As they grow older, the stutterers suffer tortures and setbacks that only dauntlessness or desperation enable them to survive. The lispers that are so numerous in certain schools are a needless retardation to the classes. (p. v)

A concern for ethical practices in speech-language pathology dates back to the 1940s. Neidecker and Blosser (1993) documented that the American Medical Association compiled a list of ethical speech correction schools and clinics for distribution to physicians in 1943. The professional services offered during the 1940s and 1950s continued to follow a medical model and focused on speech, fluency, and voice. Students were taken out of the classroom and seen individually, or in small groups, in a separate therapy room within the school. The speech correctionist conducted isolated sessions that were not at all linked to the regular classroom curriculum. Services focused on curing or eliminating the symptoms of the speech impairment. The speech correctionist wrote the program goals, selected or made therapy materials, designed the activities, established the criteria for success, measured progress, and determined dismissals from special services independently and without regard to other aspects of the student's education. The goal was to cure students of their **speech impediments**, **stammering**, and voice problems.

Before 1954, most school districts excluded any student from schooling who demonstrated cognitive abilities less than that of a 5-year-old child. Persons with moderate-to-severe cognitive disabilities, as well as children with physical disabilities, typically were discriminated against and excluded from public schools. These youths were either warehoused in large institutions or hidden in family homes, where they received no educational services and no speech-language services. Children of color and those from diverse cultures experienced similar discrimination. Freiberg (2003) described the brutal practice known as the *boarding school system*. The boarding school system began in 1878, however, by the end of the 1930s all such schools were closed in the United States. The purpose of the boarding school system was to separate Native American Indian children from their homes and communities and indoctrinate them with an "American" lifestyle. The children's cultural garb was replaced with military-style uniforms; their traditionally long hair was cut short; their religious belongings were confiscated; and they were forced to learn English through punitive means. "The boarding school system marked the most systematic assault on American Indian languages and cultures; and while the methodology gradually fell out of favor, the philosophy itself generally did not" (Freiberg, p.10).

Across the United States, students of color also were discriminated against and forced to attend segregated schools, which typically had meager budgets, inadequate materials, poorly trained teachers, and low academic expectations.

The Quiet Revolution

Equality for all children in public schools achieved a milestone in 1954, when the U.S. Supreme Court ruled in the case of *Brown v. Board of Education* that "separate but equal" is inherently unequal. *Brown v. Board of Education* spurred the Civil Rights Movement that captured the media's attention. At the same time, a less publi-

cized "quiet revolution" on behalf of people with disabilities was taking place. Lowe (1993) identified the beginning of the quiet revolution as 1961, when President John F. Kennedy called a Presidential Panel on Mental Retardation, which led to the passage of the Elementary and Secondary Education Act as Public Law (PL) 89-10 in 1965. PL 89-10 provided states with funds to evaluate and educate some, but not all, students with special needs. In 1966, the Bureau of Education for the Handicapped (BEH) was created, and model demonstration programs for the education of children with disabilities were funded by the Handicapped Children's Early Education Act (PL 90-247).

Three early court cases in this era heavily influenced public school services for children with disabilities. The first was *Brown v. Board of Education*. The second occurred in 1971, when the Supreme Court ruled in the *Pennsylvania Association for Retarded Children v. Commonwealth of Pennsylvania* case that it was not legal to refuse to educate children who had mental ages of less than 5 years. The third famous case occurred in 1972, when the court ruled in *Mills v. D.C. Board of Education* that public schools could not use the excuse of inadequate resources as a reason to deny students with disabilities an education.

Freiberg (2003) documented that the Title VI of the Civil Rights Act of 1964, the Bilingual Education Act of 1968, and the Equal Education Opportunity Act of 1974 shaped America's public education system for children of color. Additional landmark judicial actions such as *Arreola v. Board of Education* (California, 1968), *Lau v. Nichols* (California, 1974), *Diana v. The State Board of Education* (California, 1970), and *Guadalupe v. Tempe Elementary School District* (California, 1972) showed that biased assessments led to enrollment of a disproportionate number of minorities in special education programs. These judicial actions also revealed that many standardized testing procedures were racially, culturally, and linguistically discriminatory, and that the practice of placing English language learners in regular classrooms without assistance was unconstitutional. Important executive actions helped provide direction for educational agencies and parents; clarified the legal rights of people with disabilities and persons who are linguistically and culturally diverse; defined bilingual programs; and established eligibility criteria for state assistance. As an example of such remedial legislation, the acts identified by Freiberg (2003) as landmark judicial acts for Native American Indian children are summarized in Table 1–1.

Other executive actions that contributed to these premises include development and publication of the U.S. Department of Health, Education, and Welfare Policy Guideline *Identification of Discrimination* (1979), the Lau Remedies issued by the Office for Civil Rights (1975), the *U.S. Code of Federal Regulations*, Number 34, Part 300.532 (a) (1973) Regs CFR0er (1999), and the bilingual-bicultural education legislation, Subchapter VII.

The extent and types of educational services offered to students with disabilities varied dra-matically from state to state. Two federal laws were passed to rectify such inequities. Moore-Brown and Montgomery (2001) documented that Congress passed the Education of the Handicapped Act (EHA) (PL 91-230) in 1970, which established minimum requirements that states must follow in order to receive federal assistance. The second important law was Section 504 of PL 93-112, passed in 1973, which served as a civil rights statement for persons with disabilities. It guaranteed that persons with disabilities, no matter which state they lived in, had the right to vote, to be educated, to be employed, and to have access to all public buildings and environments open to the general public.

In 1975, President Gerald Ford signed into law PL 94-142, known as the Education for All Handicapped Children Act. PL 94-142 and its subsequent amendments shaped an entirely new educational experience for children with disabilities

Table 1–1. Key Legislation Supporting the Unique Needs of Native American Indian Children

Act	Year	Relevance	Public Law
Indian Education Act	1972	Provided supplemental funds for urban and reservation schools in response to the Kennedy Report, which found that such schools were doing an inadequate job of educating children from Native American Indian cultures.	
Indian Self-Determination and Education Assistance Act	1978	Defined tribal sovereignty (the right of tribes to manage their own affairs without the interference of federal, state, or outside influence). This law gave tribes the right to self-govern, determine the use of their resources, and build their community infrastructure.	PL 93-638
American Indian Religious Freedom Act	1978	Ensured that Native American Indian people, like other Americans, have the right and privilege to practice their tribal religions without fear of alienation or discrimination.	PL 95-341
Indian Child Welfare Act	1978	Protected Native American Indian children from being taken from their families. When a child was brought into the social services system, this act ensured that Native American Indian parents and members of the extended family had the first opportunity to exercise custodial rights.	PL 96-608

Source: Freiberg (2003).

(Lowe, 1993). The educational mandates set forth in PL 94-142 as described by Lowe are summarized here:

- Students with disabilities were guaranteed a free, appropriate public education and all of the related services they needed to benefit from that education.
- Every student, no matter how profound the disability, had to be served with no cost to the family.
- States had to have a "child find" program for identifying students with disabilities.
- Every student was entitled to a nonbiased evaluation and appropriate placement.
- The rights of the students and their parents were protected through legal due process.
- The federal government promised funds for state and local agencies to carry out educational programs.
- Provisions were made for the monitoring and evaluation of educational programs.
- Educational programs had to be individualized to meet the needs of the student.
- An **individualized education program** (**IEP**) had to be created for each student, to serve as a process and as a record to meet that student's goals.
- Parents and legal guardians were given the right to question activities they might regard as discriminatory, inappropriate, or unfair.
- Parents, legal guardians, or appointed surrogates had to be informed, in writing, of every change before it was proposed or discussed.
- Parents, legal guardians, or appointed surrogates had to be actively involved in decision making and in the writing of the IEP document.
- Students with disabilities had to be educated with their nondisabled peers to the greatest extent possible.

- The terms *deaf*, *deaf-blind*, *hard-of-hearing*, *mentally retarded*, *multi-handicapped*, *orthopedically impaired*, *other health impaired*, *seriously emotionally disturbed*, *specific learning disability*, *visually handicapped*, and *communication disability* were specifically defined.

The definition of a communication disability included in PL 94-142 shifted school-based speech-language services from the auspices of regular education into the category of special education. The alignment of speech-language services with special education heavily influenced the roles and responsibilities of school-based **speech-language pathologists** (SLPs).

In 1986, President Ronald Reagan signed into law PL 99-457. Neidecker and Bloser (1993) identified five major changes to PL 94-142 that were incorporated into PL 99-457, as follows:

1. Funds were provided to states that wanted to establish programs for children with disabilities from birth to the age of 2 years.
2. Educators had to design **individualized family service plans** (IFSPs) for services involving children between the ages of birth through 2 years.
3. Financial support was increased for states to provide services for children with disabilities from the ages of 3 to 5 years.
4. Discretionary programs for personnel training, programs for children with severe disabilities, research, and demonstration projects were reauthorized.
5. Services had to be provided by qualified personnel. All service providers in the schools had to meet the highest requirements in each state for that discipline. This meant that in Wisconsin, as well as in many other states, school-based SLPs had to have a master's degree.

In 1988, Congress passed the Technology-Related Assistance for Individuals with Disabilities Act (PL 100-407) and that research and development funded by PL 94-142, PL 99-457, and

PL 100-407 resulted in a dramatic shift in the philosophy of education related to individuals with disabilities (Lowe, 1993). The medical model and idea of "curing" students of their disability was replaced with a **cognitive-developmental model.** The cognitive-developmental model fostered the notion that educators must work as a team to help build on the strengths of an individual student in order to remediate his or her weaknesses. The therapeutic focus broadened to incorporate modifications to the educational environment and modifications to the teaching styles, as well as interventions to address the needs of the individual student. This new philosophy required collaboration among all educators. Speech correctionists became known as "speech-language clinicians" and later as SLPs. The age-old practice of conducting services in isolated rooms focused on isolated goals, unique materials, and criteria devoid of the general curriculum was slowly replaced with collaborative service delivery models employed in the **least restrictive environment.** Providing speech-language services while using regular education course content, writing curriculum-based goals, and incorporating curriculum-based materials began to evolve.

Movement Toward Inclusion

In 1990, all of the amendments to PL 94-142 and some new revisions were incorporated into one law, the Individuals with Disabilities Education Act (IDEA). The title of this law reflected the American Psychological Association's guidelines for "people first" language. Such language advocated for the dignity of the individual by not defining a person by his or her disability (Moore-Brown & Montgomery, 2001). For example, instead of the term *retarded child*, use of the term *child with a cognitive disability* was advocated.

Supreme Court rulings continued to shape the equality and quality of special educational services. In 1993, the court ruled in *Oberti v. Board of Education of Borough of Clementon School District* that lack of teacher training was not a reason to exclude a student with a disability

from the regular education classroom. In 1996, the court ruled in *Daniel R.R. v. State Board of Education* that the school must determine whether placement in the regular classroom, with supplementary services, can be achieved satisfactorily before an alternative special education classroom was offered.

In 1997, IDEA was reauthorized with the intent of improving the educational performance of students with disabilities by providing them with greater access to the general education curriculum. More emphasis was placed on the meaning of *least restrictive environment.* The mandate of IDEA '97 went beyond what was then known as **mainstreaming.** Mainstreaming reflected the attitude that students with disabilities had to earn the privilege to participate in the general education classroom by demonstrating progress on IEP goals and showing they were ready to be included. IDEA '97 clarified that it was the right of students with disabilities to be educated with nondisabled peers to the maximum extent possible in the least restrictive environment, which was defined as the general education classroom. With IDEA '97, educators were challenged with bringing special education and support services to students in the classroom, rather than pulling students out of the classroom and providing services in isolated settings. IDEA '97 mandated **inclusive practices**, not just mainstreaming. The success of inclusive practices required even greater communication among school administrators, general education teachers, special education teachers, support personnel, and parents or legal guardians.

Decreased school dropout rates, successful transitions from school to community; proactive approaches to students' behavioral problems, and recognition of parents as equal partners in the assessment, evaluation, and IEP processes were additional advances that resulted from IDEA '97 (Moore-Brown & Montgomery, 2001). Adequate federal funding, however, proved to be one of the greatest challenges related to the execution of all these mandates. As documented by Schraeder (2001), when PL 94-142 was authorized in 1975, the federal government was supposed to pay 40% of the costs of all special education and related services. In reality, federal funding reached only approximately 15%, forcing local school districts to spend more of the general education budget on special education services.

The lack of federal funding for special education and related services often pitted general education and special education services against each other at the local level. Local school boards had to make difficult decisions about where local tax dollars would be used. Local school districts facing the mandate of inclusive practices had to start examining the practical issues involved, such as those identified by Burnette (1996). Burnette's relevant questions are summarized as follows:

- Are there enough resources to provide adequate aids, support, related services and accommodations tailored to each individual?
- Is the school building accessible and of physical barriers?
- Do educators have time set aside for solving problems, planning, collaboration, and group discussion?
- Is it possible to keep the staff-to-student ratio low?
- Does the school atmosphere celebrate diversity?
- Does the curriculum allow for the diverse needs of students?
- Does the school environment and curriculum foster student interactions and peer support?
- Are educators properly trained to provide an inclusive setting and also address conflict resolution?
- Does the school district provide staff development?
- Does the school provide specialized support systems and personnel?

Institutions of higher education also were challenged to keep pace with the evolving mandates of the federal laws. General educators claimed that they had not been adequately trained to deal with students with disabilities. Likewise, special educators, SLPs, occupational therapists, and physical therapists were reluctant to give up their isolated therapy rooms, which appeared to be more conducive to the students' individualized learning. Nevertheless, parent advocates continued to push for inclusive practices, with the vision of their children's "fitting in" and becoming productive members of society. Gradually, more effective inclusive practices were developed through collaborative efforts between general educators, special educators, support services, the community of learners, parents and legal guardians, and local businesses. Ehren (2000) cautioned that school-based SLPs must avoid becoming tutors. A remediation focus must be maintained when inclusive practices are used. The IEP team needs to focus on what it is that makes the SLP uniquely trained to conduct this educational activity that no other educator or program assistant has the knowledge, skills, or dispositions to execute.

Inclusive Practices and Accountability

The No Child Left Behind Act (NCLB) of 2002 placed a strong emphasis on accountability. The President's Commission on Excellence in Special Education (PCESE, 2002) described the purpose of NCLB: "On January 8, 2002, President George W. Bush signed the *No Child Left Behind Act* into law. . . . We became a nation committed to judging the schools by one measure and one measure alone: whether every boy and every girl is learning— regardless of race, family background or disability status" (p. 1). The National Center on Educational Outcomes (NCEO, 2002 applauded NCLB because it required students with disabilities to reach high academic standards. NCLB contained four basic education reform principles: (1) accountability, (2) increased flexibility and local control, (3) strengthening teacher quality, and (4) evidence-based practice.

Accountability

Before NCLB, students with disabilities often were excluded from statewide and districtwide assessments. Local school boards typically used those assessment results to identify the district's strengths, challenges, and needs and created school district policies accordingly. Parents of students with disabilities were concerned that the needs of their children and adolescents were being ignored in this important policy-making procedure because students with disabilities were being excluded from the assessment process. NCLB held schools accountable for the educational achievement of students with and without disabilities by requiring all students to participate in assessment programs. As a result of the NCLB mandates, school-based SLPs began to collaborate on an educational team to create assessment accommodations and alternative assessment tools, as needed, that allowed students with disabilities to participate in the statewide and districtwide assessments. As stated by the IDEA Partnership (2000), assessment accommodations were defined as an alteration in the way a test is administered or the way a student takes a test. Such accommodations, however, do not alter the content of the test or the performance expectation. Five types of assessment accommodations defined by the IDEA Partnership are summarized in Table 1–2.

The types of accommodations allowed on statewide tests may vary from state to state. State departments of public instruction provide guidelines regarding the type of accommodations allowed.

NCLB also influenced the way IEPs were written. In the post-NCLB era, IEP goals were written in language that reflected the academic content standards established by each state. The academic content standards define what all students should know and be able to do to be considered proficient at each grade level. NCLB introduced the concept of **adequate yearly progress** (AYP). Each state was required to identify the regular incremental improvement required from year to year, with all students reaching a proficient status within 12 years, by the 2013–2014 academic year. The results of state assessments for students with disabilities must be included in the determination of AYP, along with the results of all other students, but also must be considered separately.

Table 1–2. Assessment Accommodations

Accommodation	Definition	Example
Timing	Changes in the duration of the testing	A child may need extended time to complete the test, or the test may be broken up into smaller units to match the child's endurance level.
Scheduling	Changes in when the testing occurs	A student may need to take the test at a different time of the day because of medication schedules that interfere with performance.
Setting	Changes in where the assessment is given	The student may be allowed to take the test in a study carrel, rather than in an open classroom.
Presentation	Changes in how an assessment is given	The test may need to be provided in Braille, or key words or phrases in the directions may need to be highlighted. Using larger print or reading the directions out loud to the child also may be required.
Response	Changes in how a student responds to an assessment	The student may be allowed to write an answer on special paper with guidelines or to point to an answer, rather than filling in a bubble-sheet, or may be permitted to use a computer or assistive technology to respond.

Source: IDEA Partnership (2000).

This separate consideration is called **disaggregated results** for the disability subgroup. Similar disaggregated results are required for English language learners (ELLs), for students from families of low socioeconomic status, and for various ethnic groups. Every group of students, however, must demonstrate adequate progress if the school as a whole is to make its AYP target. Schools that do not meet AYP targets suffer adverse consequences (NCEO, 2002).

Increased Flexibility and Local Control

The IDEA legislation moved children with disabilities out of institutions and into classrooms and from the outskirts of society to the center of focus in education. Unfortunately, IDEA also required excessive paperwork and meticulous documentation of procedures. The spirit of NCLB was to place more emphasis on student outcomes based on AYP, rather than focusing on documentation related to due process, procedural safeguards, and parents' rights. NCLB allowed schools to spend up to half of their federal education dollars based on local needs, rather than on the federal programs (e.g., Title I, Safe and Drug-Free Schools, Teacher Quality State Grants, Educational Technology, Innovative Programs) for which those dollars were originally earmarked (NCEO, 2002).

Parental Choice

NCLB advocated giving parents the choice to remove their students from schools that were not meeting AYP to schools that were higher-performing. NCLB also advocated giving parents the choice to remove students from unsafe schools to safer schools. The idea of giving parents school vouchers to remove their students from public schools and enroll them in private or parochial schools gained momentum through NCLB.

Highly Qualified Teachers

The PCESE (2002) noted that many students in America were being placed in special education programs because they were not able to read. The commission questioned whether such placements resulted from true disabilities or from inadequate teaching. NCLB mandated that public schools hire only qualified teachers for Title I –supported programs as of the 2002–2003 school year and develop a plan to have all teachers be highly qualified by the end of the 2005–2006 school year (Ruesch, 2004). NCLB left it up to each state, however, to define what is meant by "highly qualified."

Evidence-Based Practice

The NCLB act required that all school districts use only those teaching strategies that are rooted in scientifically based research. According to Ruesch (2004), the term *scientifically based research* embodies the following:

- Research that involves the application of rigorous, systematic, and objective procedures to obtain reliable and valid knowledge relevant to education activities and programs and includes research that:
- Employs systematic, empirical methods that draw on observation or experiment
- Involves rigorous data analyses that are adequate to test the stated hypotheses and justify the general conclusions drawn
- Relies on measurements or observational methods that provide reliable and valid data across evaluators and observers, across multiple measurements and observations, and across studies by the same or different investigators
- Is evaluated using experimental or quasiexperimental designs in which individuals, entities, programs, or activities are assigned to different conditions and with a preference for random-assignment experiments, or other designs to the extent that those designs contain within-condition or across-condition controls

■ Ensures that experimental studies are presented in sufficient detail and clarity to allow for replication or, at a minimum, offer the opportunity to build systematically on their findings

■ Has been accepted by a peer-reviewed journal or approved by a panel of independent experts through a comparably rigorous, objective, and scientific review [Section 9101(37), Individuals with Disabilities Education Improvement Act (IDEA, 2004)]

Individuals with Disabilities Education Improvement Act

President George W. Bush signed the **Individuals with Disabilities Education Improvement Act** into law on December 3, 2004, so the law became known as **IDEA '04**. (Even though the acronym for the law technically should be IDEIA, the well-known acronym IDEA is still used in referring to the reauthorized law.) The law consisted of five parts; Parts A, B, C, and subpart I of Part D took effect on July 1, 2005. IDEA '04 addressed six major concepts: (1) paperwork reduction (including changes in the IEP), (2) qualified provider, (3) early intervention, (4) transitions, (5) research and development, and (6) funding. The six major characteristics of the changes incorporated into IDEA '04 as identified by ASHA (2004) are summarized next.

Paperwork Reduction

Based on a report by the PCESE (2002), excessive paperwork was one of the major concerns that surfaced under IDEA '97. Too much time was being spent on documentation and not enough time was being spent on the actual education of students with disabilities. It was questioned whether or not the burdensome paperwork actually translated into educational benefits. For example, one school district estimated that under IDEA '97, the addition of one student to the case-load of a school-based SLP resulted in an additional 10 meetings and 52 forms (ASHA, 2002). In hopes of maximizing the use of resources for the best interest of students, IDEA '04 allowed waivers of statutory or regulatory requirements under Part B in up to 15 states for up to 4 years. The purpose of the waivers was to allow those states to develop pilot projects for alternative, more efficient paperwork. The waivers did not grant the pilot projects freedom to ignore the right of a student with a disability to receive a free and appropriate public education in the least restrictive environment or the due process rights of parents and legal guardians. The effectiveness of the waivers and any recommendations for their broader implementation had to be carefully scrutinized by the Secretary of the U.S. Department of Education and reported annually to Congress. IDEA '04 eliminated the need for short-term objectives or benchmarks in the IEP for most students. Short-term objectives or benchmarks were necessary only if the student participates in alternative assessments aligned to alternative educational standards. IDEA '04 required the Secretary of Education to publish and disseminate forms for a model IEP, IFSP, notice of procedural safeguards, and prior written notices. IDEA '04 also allowed a member of the IEP team to be excused from an IEP meeting under three circumstances: (1) if no modifications were being made to that member's area of curriculum or service, (2) if the member provided input before the meeting, and (3) if all of the other IEP team members agreed to the member's excusal before the meeting. IDEA '04 permitted LEAs to consolidate IEP meetings and reevaluation meetings; allowed parents to participate in IEP team and placement meetings via videoconferences or teleconference calls; allowed modifications to be made to the student's current IEP without having to convene an IEP meeting; and allowed a three-year IEP for students 18 years of age and older.

Qualified Provider

IDEA '97 did not define the term **highest qualified provider** and left that definition up to each state. Most states adopted the definition of a qualified provider as a person licensed in the area of exceptionality. Some states interpreted the law as allowing a person with a **para-educator** license to function independently in the same capacity as that of a fully certified SLP. A para-educator is a person who has acquired an associate's degree from a 2-year technical school. So long as the para-educator held a state license, the letter of the law was met. When NCLB was authorized mandating highly qualified educators, it was expected that IDEA '04 would follow with a clear definition of the term. That outcome did not come about.

Early Intervention

The IQ discrepancy formula that existed under IDEA '97 required a student to fail academically before eligibility criteria for a learning disability were met. IDEA '04 eliminated the IQ discrepancy requirement. As a way to advocate for early intervention, IDEA '04 allowed schools to use up to 15% of its federal dollars for supportive services to help students not yet identified as having disabilities, but who required additional academic and behavioral supports to succeed in the general education environment. IDEA '04 encouraged schools that showed a disproportionate number of students of color enrolled in special education to strengthen their prereferral system.

Transitions

IDEA '04 allowed parents of children in "birth-to-three" programs the option to delay enrollment of a free and appropriate public education so that the child could remain in that program if the IFSP included an educational component that promoted school readiness and incorporated preliteracy, language, and numeric skills. This change allowed participating states to combine early intervention and preschool programs to better serve families of children with special needs and to use Part B and Part C monies to do so. When a child exited from a Part C (birth-to-three) program, the IFSP had to include a description of the transition services. Steps for exiting the Part C program had to be included in the transition plans. At the high school level, the first IEP that was in place after a student's 16th birthday had to include appropriate measurable postsecondary transition goals based on age-appropriate assessments. Those assessments had to relate to the training, education, employment, independent living skills, and transition services that an adolescent needed to reach those goals. Before IDEA '04, transition services applied to students at age 14.

Research and Development

Research formally conducted or funded by the Office of Special Education Programs (OSEP) was shifted to the Institute of Education Sciences (IES) under a new Part E in IDEA '04. Grant funding under a program called the State Personnel Preparation and Professional Development Grants gave top priority to states that had the greatest personnel shortages or demonstrated the greatest difficulty meeting Part B requirements for personnel qualifications.

Funding

IDEA '04 established a funding schedule for increasing federal dollars by approximately $2.3 billion per year for six years. If the funding schedule was honored, IDEA would achieve full funding (i.e., the 40% per pupil funding that was promised when the original law PL 94-142 was written in 1975) by the year 2011. Although IDEA '04 authorized the funding schedule, however, it was not mandatory.

Successes and Failures

The successes and failures of IDEA and NCLB may be attributed to how local school boards make decisions about funding and policy issues. There is a strong heritage of local control in the United States with respect to the quality and equality of educational practices. The work of Kozol (1967,

2005) documented some of the worst failures of the American public education system. The IDEA Partnership (2007) provided an entire library of information related to the successes and failures of IDEA and NCLB. One may find glowing examples of success or despicable examples of failures in the American education system. Addressing such inequities may be one of the greatest challenges facing educators today.

Roles and Responsibilities of Today's School-Based Speech-Language Pathologist

When speech services were first provided in schools in the early 1900s, the speech correctionist was expected to cure children of their impediments based on a medical model. The prevailing disposition toward those children was less than favorable and often demeaning. Over the years, the roles and responsibilities of the school-based SLP have been heavily influenced by mandates in local, state, and federal laws. Likewise, the dispositions toward persons with disabilities also have evolved. As proclaimed by the U.S. Congress in 1997:

> Disability is a natural part of the human experience and in no way diminishes the right of individuals to participate in or contribute to society. Improving educational results for children with disabilities is an essential element of our national policy of ensuring equality of opportunity, full participation, independent living, and economic self-sufficiency for individuals with disabilities. (U.S. Congress, 1997 [Sec. 601(c)])

ASHA (1999) supported this shift in dispositions: "A student-centered focus drives team decision-making. Comprehensive assessment and thorough evaluation provide information for appropriate eligibility, intervention, and dismissal decisions. Intervention focuses on the student's abilities, rather than disabilities. Intervention plans are consistent with current research and practice" (p. 2).

If asked, "What is it that you do in the schools?" the speech correctionist from the 1900s might have answered: "I cure children of their speech impediments so that they are neither an embarrassment to their families or themselves nor a burden on the teacher or society." If asked the same question today, the school-based SLP of the twenty-first century may answer: "I work on an educational team to encourage, educate, and enlighten students and society and to ensure that all children receive a free and appropriate public education. Our team goal is to bring individualized services and accommodations to students in the least restrictive environment while they make acceptable progress on curriculum-based standards. Our vision is that all students will ultimately become productive citizens in America's workforce as they exercise their rights to life, liberty, and the pursuit of happiness." The stark difference between these two teaching philosophies is clear. The former statement reflects the discrimination toward individuals with disabilities that was widespread during the 1900s; the latter statement reflects the modern-day movement that goes beyond inclusive practices in the new millennium. It embraces the philosophy that is advocated by the Whole Schooling Consortium (2002): "Whole Schools form a culture where all children achieve at their highest levels and where they learn and practice a socially responsible, democratic, and inclusive form of community they will carry valuably into their adult lives" (p. 1).

The complex responsibilities faced by modern-day SLPs yield equally complex roles. ASHA (1999) identified 15 roles for which the SLP may be responsible in the school setting. These roles are summarized next.

Prevention

As an active member of the educational team, the SLP is heavily involved in prevention activities. IDEA '04 mandated that all possible regular education options be exhausted before a student is referred for special education and related services. The SLP may meet with general educators and other special educators on a weekly, biweekly, or monthly basis to brainstorm regarding services and accommodations that may be tried in the general education setting. These formalized weekly meetings are held before a referral is made. Parents may be informed that a prereferral meeting is being held and may receive a copy of the prereferral plan that has been developed. The parent does not need to provide permission for such a meeting to occur, however, because it is within the realm of general education services. Behavioral contracts, youth-tutoring-youth programs, foster grandparent programs, hearing conservation environmental modifications, Title I reading and math programs, reduced class size, modified texts, and parent volunteer supports are just a few examples of regular education options that may be components of the prevention plan. A prevention plan summary may be shared with the parent and also placed in the student's cumulative file. Additional prevention team meetings may be devoted to follow-up analysis to determine if the strategies, interventions, and accommodations designed to assist the student were successful. The SLP also may engage in an information dissemination program (e.g., provide prenatal information for the prevention of fetal alcohol syndrome or provide vocal hygiene information for cheerleaders or choir members). The SLP may collaborate with the school nurse or the audiologist to conduct hearing screenings, prekindergarten screenings, or speech-language screenings. The SLP also may provide prevention consultation services regarding environmental hazards such as lead poisoning. The ASHA (2003) established professional standards for its Certificate of Clinical Competence (CCC) that include prevention. IDEA '04 strengthened the mandate for prereferral activities in hopes that the disproportionate number of students of color enrolled in special education would diminish.

Identification

The SLP is uniquely trained and qualified to determine whether a student exhibits a communicative delay, disorder, or difference. The ASHA has identified nine disorder categories: articulation, voice, fluency, swallowing, language comprehension and production, cognitive aspects of communica-

tion, social aspects of communication, phonemic-phonological aspects of communication, and hearing. IDEA '04 strengthened the mandate for "child find" efforts through screenings and information dissemination activities.

Assessment

IDEA '04 mandated that assessment data used in the IEP process be collected from a variety of sources. For example, the SLP may engage in record reviews and collection of case histories; document outcomes from prereferral plans; conduct clinical observations in classroom settings; administer standardized tests; conduct interviews of parents, teachers, peers, and others; assemble portfolios of the student's work; and complete developmental checklists. In other modes of data collection, the SLP may conduct authentic assessments, dynamic assessments, play-based assessments, functional assessments, and curriculum-based assessments; perform speech and language sample analysis; or use instrumentation specific to the field.

Evaluation

The SLP must collaborate with other members of the IEP team to interpret the assessment data that have been collected. The team must decide whether or not an eligibility criterion for one or more of the nine disorder categories has been met. The team must further determine whether or not that impairment results in a disability that warrants special education or related services. The SLP and other members of the IEP team must write a statement of the present level of educational and functional performance that reflects the student's strengths, needs (or challenges), interests, and learning style.

Development of Goals

The SLP must be familiar with the curriculum standards of the general education program so that curriculum-based, standards-based goals may be developed for each student's IEP or IFSP. The SLP must conduct a task analysis so that the goal may be achieved through developmental, sequential, or logical steps.

Caseload Management

The SLP must be aware of local, state, and federal mandates and justify all of the services that are conducted with, for, or on behalf of the students. The SLP also must know how to access the research-based evidence base for the educational practices that are used.

Intervention

The SLP must be flexible and provide a variety of service delivery options (e.g., monitor, pull-out, consultation, classroom-based, self-contained, community-based, home-based, team teach) so that a continuum of services ensure the least restrictive environment that is still appropriate for the needs of each student. These service delivery options must be applicable to all nine disorder categories. NCLB placed a greater emphasis on reading and math skills for all students. Consequently, SLPs work more closely with a team of educators to make language and literacy connections across the curriculum. The role that the SLP plays in the language and literacy connection varies from state to state. In Wisconsin, for example, SLPs do not teach reading, but they do teach the language underpinnings that facilitate literacy. In Rhode Island, however, some SLPs teach reading as part of their job description.

Counseling

The SLP must use interpersonal techniques to engage students, educators, caregivers, and parents or legal guardians in the processes of information counseling, problem solving, transitioning, cause-and-effect reasoning, carryover programming, self-help or advocacy, and self-monitoring activities.

The SLP must be able to identify behaviors that indicate the need for referrals to other human services professionals.

Reevaluation

The SLP must collect observable, measurable data to document progress based on pretestand post-test findings. The SLP must interpret the data to determine whether modifications need to be made in the IEP and whether the student is ready for either dismissal from special services or transition to another type of service delivery model.

Transition

The SLP must communicate with other agencies and other professionals to provide services in the least restrictive environment. When working with a preschool population, the SLP may go into the home or the day care setting and consult with parents or caregivers. When working with adolescents, the SLP may "job shadow" a student to analyze the communication competencies that the student must develop in order to be successful in that setting.

Dismissal

The SLP should collaborate with others when considering the dismissal of a student from special services. Observable, measurable data from a variety of sources should be collected, analyzed, interpreted, and documented.

Supervision

The SLP may agree to observe a student teacher; mentor a beginning-level educator; or provide supervision for a **clinical fellowship**. The SLP may supervise para-educators or program assistants. The SLP also may serve as an information resource specialist or liaison to other SLPs in the school district.

Documentation

The SLP conducts multiple types of documentation activities for a variety of purposes. The following list is suggestive of the wide range of such documentation activities but is not all-inclusive: third party billing, progress on IEP goals, annual yearly progress under NCLB, modified or alternative statewide or districtwide assessments, clinical observations regarding the effects of newly administered medications, district-mandated report cards, and reports written for outside agencies.

Research

The SLP may engage in action research, single-subject design research, database collection, survey analysis, or experimental designs. IDEA '04 and NCLB strengthened the need for evidence-based practice in special education and related services.

Leadership and Advocacy

The SLP has become an integral part of the school culture and often serves on leadership teams that create curriculum standards, select textbooks, execute districtwide initiatives, create proactive behavior programs, and so forth. Because the SLP typically provides individualized services for students, those students often forge a close bond with the SLP. It is not surprising that a large number of SLPs report that they are often the person that a student in need turns to when seeking help related to abuse or neglect. The SLP must know how to be a strong advocate. Advocacy also means advocating for programs and the profession.

In school districts that employ more than one SLP, it is not uncommon for role differentiation to occur. For example, one SLP may be responsible for prevention, identification, assessment, evaluation, IEP/IFSP development, and reevaluation, while other SLPs execute the other roles and responsibilities. It is rarely the case that one SLP assumes all 15 roles and responsibilities. In smaller, rural school districts, however, this may be necessary from time to time.

Requisite Knowledge for the School-Based Speech-Language Pathologist

The modern-day SLP must have a solid foundation in order to execute all of the roles and responsibilities faced in the school setting. ASHA (2003) established the **Knowledge and Skills Acquisition** (KASA) form that defines the knowledge and skills delineated in its CCC standards. The professional knowledge base defined by the ASHA KASA includes the following:

- The principles of biological sciences, physical sciences, mathematics, and social and behavioral sciences
- Basic human communication processes including biological, neurological, acoustic, psychological, developmental, linguistic, and cultural aspects
- Swallowing processes including biological, neurological, acoustic, psychological, developmental, linguistic, and cultural aspects
- The nature of speech, language, hearing, and communication disorders and differences and swallowing disorders
- The prevention of disorders or delays of articulation, fluency, voice and resonance, receptive and expressive language, hearing, swallowing, cognitive aspects of communication, social aspects of communication, and communication modalities
- Etiologies of disorders including: articulation, fluency, voice and resonance, receptive and expressive language, hearing, swallowing, cognitive aspects of communication, social aspects of communication, and communication modalities
- Characteristics of articulation, fluency, voice and resonance, receptive and expressive language, hearing, swallowing, cognitive aspects of communication, social aspects of communication, and communication modalities

- Intervention strategies for remediation of articulation, fluency, voice and resonance, receptive and expressive language, hearing, swallowing, cognitive aspects of communication, social aspects of communication, and communication modalities

Essential Skills for the School-Based Speech-Language Pathologist

The school-based SLP must know how to apply theory to practice. ASHA requires all SLPs in training to acquire a minimum of 400 clinical clock hours. Twenty-five of those hours must be in clinical observation. The remaining 375 hours must reflect the scope of practice across the lifespan. As summarized from the work of Kwiatkowski, Murray-Branch, and Schraeder (2005), the SLP must demonstrate specific clinical competencies, including the following:

- Administer, score, interpret, and make recommendations based on screening processes.
- Collect case history information.
- Select assessment models that are based on research or scientific principles related to the population served and articulate a rationale for the assessment model based on sound theoretical principles.
- Administer standardized test instruments.
- Perform systematic nonstandardized assessment, dynamic assessment, and authentic assessment.
- Conduct clinical observations.
- Accurately analyze and interpret assessment data.
- Identify the individual's strengths, challenges (needs), interests, and learning style based on the assessment data.
- Prioritize the needs of the individual and translate those needs into therapeutic goals.

- Develop a curriculum-based IEP that may be implemented in the least restrictive environment.
- Identify the most appropriate service delivery model that accommodates the individual's unique learning style.
- Select and adapt educational materials.
- Use instrumentation skillfully, when appropriate.
- Use strategies related to motivation, reinforcement, retention, and transfer of learning.
- Manage off-task behaviors using proactive strategies as well as reactive techniques.
- Collect quantitative and qualitative data.
- Interpret data to modify plans or define success.
- Schedule all workload responsibilities efficiently.
- Maintain client records.
- Create documentation using an objective, clinical writing style.
- Collaborate with parents, guardians, caregivers, and other professionals.
- Comply with policies, legal mandates, and regulations.
- Provide counseling within the scope of practice.
- Refer clients to other professionals, when appropriate.
- Practice cultural competency.
- Maintain confidentiality.

Dispositions Toward Persons with Disabilities: Considerations in Practice for the School-Based Speech-Language Pathologist

Dispositions are defined as the attitudes, proclivities, and propensities that drive one's actions. The dispositions toward persons with disabilities conveyed by Scripture in his 1912 text are very different from those conveyed by the "people first" language of 1990. Similarly, the ten guiding principles advocated by ASHA in 1999 are different from the six principles of Whole Schooling of

2005. Each set of dispositions illustrates how attitudes have changed over time. The SLP must keep abreast with the dispositions that modern-day society embraces. To do so, the SLP must become a life-long learner, critical thinker, and problem solver. If the SLP embraces these characteristics and practices them throughout a career, dispositions that reflect changing societal trends may be readily assimilated. Researchers studying effective thinking and intelligent behavior (Ennis, 1985; Feuerstein, Rand, Hoffman, & Miller, 1980; Glathorn & Baron, 1985; Perkins, 1985; Sternberg, 1984 identified 12 characteristics of an effective problem solver. According to Costa and Schraeder (1985), these characteristics are persistence, decreased impulsivity, empathy, flexibility, metacognitive reflection (**metacognition**), accuracy and precision, questioning, accommodation and assimilation, exact language and thought, use of all senses, curiosity, and creativity. Each of these characteristics is described next:

- *Persistence*. The effective, efficient problem solver is always looking for ways to expand his or her bag of tricks. The question "What else might work?" is always on the mind of the SLP. Clinical competence requires a systematic approach to assessment, task analysis, data collection, and evaluation. The persistent SLP would rather discover three ways to solve one problem than be limited in knowing only one way to solve three problems.
- *Decreased impulsivity*. The SLP often must inhibit the first idea that comes to mind. Considering alternatives is an art that must be nurtured over time. Applying the science of clarifying goals, planning strategies, respecting cultural diversity, and considering consequences will decrease the amount of trial and error.
- *Empathy*. Empathy has been identified as the highest form of intelligent behavior. Piaget called it overcoming egocentrism. The SLP must work toward the ability to paraphrase another person's ideas, detect feelings or emotions, and express anther person's concepts in a nonjudgmental manner. The empathic SLP understands the fear of the disfluent speaker, the frustration of the adult with developmental disabilities, and the exasperation of the child with a **neurogenic speech disorder**.
- *Flexibility*. The school-based SLP must collaborate with others. Collaboration is possible only when the SLP remains flexible and open to new ideas and new approaches that are evidence based.
- *Metacognition*. The effective problem solver is able to self-reflect and understand his or her own line of thinking. The SLP must be able to objectively evaluate personal issues of culture, strengths, challenges, and learning style.
- *Accuracy and precision*. The school-based SLP must know how to collect data in objective, measurable terms. Clinical competence requires clarity.
- *Questioning*. The school-based SLP must know how to find problems as well as how to solve problems. Divergent thinking is as valuable as convergent thinking. The SLP knows that the best answer to a question often is another thoughtful question.
- *Accommodation and assimilation*. The SLP must know how to draw upon past knowledge and apply it to new situations. The SLP effectively uses foresight and hindsight to assess, self-reflect, form associations, and identify critical attributes relevant to important situations.
- *Exact language and thought*. The SLP must know how to create criteria and articulate supportive evidence using specific language. Clinical competence requires the ability to use exact terms and synthesize information into operationally defined sequences or hierarchies.

- *Use of all senses.* To know a goal, it must be envisioned. The SLP must know how to scrutinize all sensory input as data are gathered, manipulated, illustrated, and analyzed.
- *Curiosity.* The SLP must enjoy the problem-solving process. Curiosity should become stronger as the problem becomes more complex. Clinical competence requires cognizant, compassionate behaviors as difficult cases are approached.
- *Creativity.* The SLP must seek feedback and be open to criticism. The SLP must strive for greater fluency, elaboration, novelty, perfection, and balance. Clinical competence requires the willingness to take risks and test limits.

Summary

Speech and language services first emerged in American public schools in the early 1900s following a movement for social justice and significant changes to child labor laws on a national level. Those services, however, were available only to students in the mainstream of society. Students with more severe disabilities, students from diverse backgrounds, and students of color generally were excluded or separated from public schools. From the 1900s to 1960s, a medical model implemented by speech correctionists was typically conducted in isolated, itinerant settings. Those services focused on speech impediments, voice problems, and stammering. A second movement of social justice came after *Brown v. the Board of Education.* As a result of the Civil Rights Movement, public school services for students from diverse backgrounds, students of color, and students with disabilities dramatically expanded. Court cases changed service delivery models. During the 1970s, research and evidence-based practices placed more emphasis on the benefits of early intervention. New service delivery models that were collaborative in nature became evident during the 1980s and 1990s. Inclusive practices, "whole schooling" philosophies, professional collaboration, curriculum-based services, curriculum-based educational standards, a focus on literacy, and increased accountability appear to be the predominant forces shaping the new millennium. From the inception of the Education of Handicapped Children Act of 1975 through IDEA '04, inadequate federal funding has been a major challenge. Nevertheless, educational practices, as well as the roles and responsibilities of the school-based SLP, have been heavily influenced by federal mandates.

Questions for Application and Review

1. Describe the possible educational experiences of a student who has been diagnosed with moderate cerebral palsy, a mild cognitive disability, delayed expressive language, and a moderate articulation disorder and whose birth date is 10/11/50.
2. Describe the possible educational experiences of a student who has been diagnosed with moderate cerebral palsy, a mild cognitive disability, delayed expressive language, and a moderate articulation disorder and whose birth date is 6/22/77.
3. Describe the possible educational experiences of a student who has been diagnosed with moderate cerebral palsy, a mild cognitive disability, delayed expressive language, and a moderate articulation disorder and whose birth date is 9/19/91.
4. Describe the possible educational experiences of a student who has been diagnosed with moderate cerebral palsy, a mild cognitive disability, delayed expressive language, and a moderate articulation disorder and whose birth date is 7/18/05.
5. Summarize the dispositions conveyed in the excerpt from Scripture's book, written in 1912?
6. What is your opinion of the dispositions conveyed in the ten guiding principles developed by ASHA in 1999 related to the roles and responsibilities of the school-based SLP?

7. What is meant by "equality and quality" in education for persons with disabilities?
8. How has NCLB shaped school-based speech-language pathology services?
9. How will IDEA '04 shape school-based speech-language pathology services in the future?
10. In your opinion, what continue to be the greatest challenges that provide roadblocks to ensuring equality and quality in public school speech-language pathology services?

References

American Speech-Language-Hearing Association. (1999). *Guidelines for the roles and responsibilities of the school-based speech-language pathologist*. Available from www.asha.org/policy

American Speech-Language-Hearing Association. (2002). *A workload analysis approach for establishing caseload standards in schools*. Rockville, MD: Author.

American Speech-Language-Hearing Association. (2003). *Knowledge and skills acquisition (KASA) summary form for certification in speech-language pathology*. Available from www.asha.org/policy

Burnette, J. (1996). Including students with disabilities in general education classrooms: From policy to practice. *The Eric Review*, *4*(3), 2–11.

Changes in IDEA 2004. (2006, Oct. 17). *The ASHA Leader*, *11*(14), 17. Retrieved December 11, 2007 from http://www.asha.org/about/publications/leaderonline/archives/2006/061017/f061017d1.htm

Costa, A., & Schraeder, T. (1989). In search of clinical competence: Strategies for success. In K. Carlson & T. Schraeder (Eds.), *A manual for clinical practicum* (pp. 1–2). Madison, WI: Authors.

Ehren, B. (2000). Maintaining a therapeutic focus and sharing responsibility for student success: Keys to in-classroom speech-language services. *Language, Speech, and Hearing Services in Schools*, *31*, 219–229.

Ennis, R. (1985). Goals for a critical thinking curriculum. In A. Costa (Ed.), *Developing minds: A resource book for teaching thinking* (pp. 68–72). Alexandria, VA: Association for Supervision and Curriculum Development.

Feuerstein, R., Rand, Y., Hoffman, M., & Miller, R. (1980). *Instrumental enrichment: An intervention program for cognitive modifiability*. Baltimore: University Park Press.

Freiberg, C. (2003). *Linguistically culturally diverse populations: American Indian and Spanish speaking*. Madison, WI: Wisconsin Department of Public Instruction.

Glatthorn, A., & Baron, J. (1985). The good thinker. In A. Costa (Ed.), *Developing minds: A resource book for teaching thinking* (pp. 49–53). Alexandria, VA: Association for Supervision and Curriculum Development.

The History Place. (1998). *Child labor in America: 1908–1912*. Retrieved January 19, 2005, from http://www.historyplace.com/unitedstates/childlabor/about.htm

IDEA Partnership. (2000). *Making assessment accommodations*. Reston, VA: Council for Exceptional Children.

IDEA Partnership. (2007). *Results for kids*. Retrieved August 18, 2007, from www.ideapartnerships.org

Kozol, J. (1967). *Death at an early age*. New York: Random House.

Kozol, J. (2005). *The shame of the nation*. New York: Random House.

Kwiatkowski, J., Murray-Branch, J., & Schraeder, T. (2005). *Clinical skills learner outcome tracking system*. Unpublished assessment tool, University of Wisconsin at Madison, Madison, WI.

Lowe, R. (1993) *Speech-language pathology and related professions in the schools*. Boston: Allyn & Bacon.

Moore-Brown, B., & Montgomery, J. (2001). *Making a difference for America's children*. Eau Claire, WI: Thinking Publications.

National Center on Educational Outcomes. (2002). Retrieved January 20, 2005 from http://education.umn.edu/NCEO/Default.html

Neidecker, E. & Blosser, J. (1993). *School programs in speech-language* (3rd ed., pp. 4–5). Englewood Cliffs, NJ: Prentice Hall.

Perkins, D. (1985). What creative thinking is. In Costa, A. (Ed.), *Developing your repertoire of teaching strategies* (pp 29–30). Alexandria, VA: Author.

President's Commission on Excellence in Special Education. (2002). Retrieved January 19, 2005, from http://www.ed.gov/inits/commissionsboards/whspecialeducation/index

Ruesch, G. (2004). *No Child Left Behind*. Paper presented at the Wisconsin Speech-Language Pathology and Audiology Association Annual Convention, April 16, 2004, Green Bay, WI.

President's Commission on Excellence in Special Education. (2002). Retrieved January 19, 2005, from http://www.ed.gov/inits/commissionsboards/whspecialeducation/index

Schraeder, T. (2001). Three current hot issues related to professional ethics. *ASHA School-Based Issues*, *2*(1), 28–30.

Scripture, E. W. (1912). *Stuttering and lisping* (p. v). New York: Macmillan.

Sternberg, R. (1984). *Beyond I.Q.: A triarchic theory of human intelligence*. New York: Cambridge University Press.

Taylor, J. (1992. Speech-language pathology services in schools (2nd ed., p. 4). Boston: Allyn & Bacon.

The History Place: Child labor in America: 1908–2005, from http://www.historyplace.com/unitedstates/childlabor/about/htm

U.S. Congress Individuals with Disabilities Education Act (2007). Title 20; Chapter 33; Subchapter I; 1400.

Whole Schooling Consortium. (2002). Retrieved January 19, 2005, from www.wholeschooling.net

Chapter 2

A WORKLOAD ANALYSIS APPROACH TO CASELOAD STANDARDS IN SCHOOLS

RELATED VOCABULARY

auditory comprehension The ability to localize, attend to, discriminate, understand, and remember oral language that is heard.

caseload The number of students who receive services from a speech-language pathologist through a variety of delivery models.

case manager The professional who manages all aspects of the IEP process on behalf of a student, conducts all relevant communications, maintains required legal documentation, and facilitates meetings.

compensation language Language written into the master contract between a school district and its employees that allows for payment of additional monies when the workload exceeds the terms agreed on within the master contract with respect to wages, hours, and working conditions.

complementary teaching A team teaching service delivery mode in which both partners teach in the classroom from their own areas of

Acknowledgement. Much of the information presented in this chapter has been condensed or adapted from the following two documents published by the American Speech-Language-Hearing Association (ASHA):

A Workload Analysis Approach to Caseload Standards in Schools. Position Statement, Technical Report, and Guidelines (ASHA, 2002)

Implementation Guide: A Workload Analysis Approach for Establishing Caseload Standards in Schools (ASHA, 2003)

Permission to publish this information has been granted. The members of the ASHA ad hoc committee that authored these two documents are Frank Cirrin and Ann Bird, co-chairs, and, in alphabetical order, Larry Biehl, Sally Disney, Ellen Estomin, Judy Rudebusch, Trici Schraeder, and Kathleen Whitmire (ex officio).

expertise. They share responsibilities for planning the program, teaching the lessons, monitoring the progress of the students, and making decisions about modifying the program.

consultation/consultative intervention A team teaching service delivery model in which the speech-language pathologist or special educator offers ideas to the regular educator or parent tailored specifically to an individual student's needs in order to maximize a student's learning or communication competence.

diagnostician A professional whose primary purpose is to conduct and/or collect assessment data for the purposes of identifying and distinguishing the difference between an impairment, delay, disorder, or difference.

direct services Speech-language intervention services provided by the speech-language pathologist directly to a student or group of students.

diversified roles Describing the delivery of speech-language services by dividing professional activities, within the scope of practice, between two or more speech-language pathologists.

expressive language The use of a rule-governed symbolic system to convey one's thoughts, feelings, desires, needs, experiences, or intentions.

free and appropriate public education (FAPE) The mandate in IDEA that public school districts must offer every child with a disability special education and related services at no additional cost to the parents or legal guardians.

indirect services All of the services that are provided for and on behalf of the student with a disability that are necessary to a free and appropriate public education.

individual family service plan (IFSP) A process and a product that guides early intervention for children with disabilities, aged birth to three, and their families. The IFSP is the means by which early intervention outcomes are implemented as mandated by Part C of the Individuals with Disabilities Education Improvement Act of 2004 (IDEA).

least restrictive environment (LRE) The mandate in IDEA that requires children with disabilities to be educated to the maximum extent possible with children who are not disabled.

metacognitive Referring to awareness of one's own thought processes and problem solving strategies as well as how they are executed. Knowing how and when one learns information as well as when and what to remember or how to organize it.

National Outcomes Measurement System (NOMS)   A national outcomes database created by the American Speech-Language-Hearing Association for speech-language pathologists and audiologists.

program support teachers   Fully certified speech-language pathologists who offer field related information, guidance, supervision, or assistance to other speech-language pathologists serving a school district or area.

receptive vocabulary   The repertoire of words and phrases that are understood.

resource room   A service delivery model in which the speech-language pathologist or special educator integrates the individualized education program goals into curriculum-based support as the students complete homework assignments in a specially designed learning environment.

speech club   A service delivery model in which the speech-language pathologist monitors how well the student with a disability is able to carry over his or her goals into unstructured, social environments with other children who are not disabled.

supportive teaching   A service delivery model in which the speech-language pathologist provides supplemental information related to the information that the regular education teacher has introduced.

teaming for reading   A service delivery model in which the speech-language pathologist collaborates with other educators to provide a comprehensive literacy program for children with disabilities and their nondisabled peers.

team teaching   A service delivery model in which the speech-language pathologist and a regular education teacher share all the roles and responsibilities related to the educational process.

utterance   A single unit of verbal expression such as a phrase or sentence.

weighted formula   A way of calculating the time intensity of tasks.

workload   All of those professional activities that a professional does with, for, and on behalf of students on a caseload that are mandated by law.

workload week   One week out of a set of weeks during which the professional conducts indirect services for or on behalf of students on a caseload, rather than providing direct intervention with the students.

Introduction

The number of children seen by any single school-based speech-language pathologist (SLP) within a work week has been a controversial issue ever since 1975, when Public Law (PL) 94-142 identified speech-language services under the auspices of special education (ASHA, 1984, 1993a, 2000a, 2002, 2003; Chiang & Rylance, 2000; Whitmire, 2000). As documented by the ASHA (2002), between 1990 and 1999, the number of children with speech-language impairments has grown by more than 10%. SLPs serve students in most other disability categories as well, all of which have shown large increases in the past 10 years (U.S. Department of Education, 2000).

As revealed by the ASHA Schools Survey (ASHA, 2004), the average caseload size remains at 50, with no differentiation among rural, suburban, and metropolitan schools. A slight variation was observed in geographical areas, however. In the northeastern area of the country, the average caseload size was 41; in the Midwest, the average caseload size was 49; and in the southern and western regions of the nation, the average caseload size was the highest at 50.

School-based SLPs must be concerned about caseload size not just in their own interest but also for the sake of the children and youth who receive their services. In 1993, the ASHA recommended that under no circumstances should a school-based SLP's caseload exceed 40, yet in 2004 the average caseload size across the United States remained at 50 (ASHA, 2004). The ASHA 1993 recommendation appeared to have been ignored for over a decade. Worse yet, some states interpreted the maximum of 40 to mean a minimum. SLPs in those states faced reductions in their contract time when their caseload sizes dipped below 40. State and local policies on caseloads for SLPs were as variable as caseload and class size regulations for other special education services. As documented by Rylance, Chiang, Russ, and Dobbs-Whitcome (1999), 28 states established maximum caseload guidelines for school SLPs, but 22 states left the power of determining caseload size up to local districts. For states with numerical guidelines,

speech-language caseload limits extended from a low of 40 in Hawaii and Wisconsin to a high of 80 in Ohio and 90 in Pennsylvania (Chiang & Rylance, 2000). The ASHA Special Interest Division for School-Based Issues contacted all state education agencies to determine current caseload sizes (ASHA, 2000e). Of the states indicating that they have established caseload caps, the maximum numbers reported ranged from 30 to 80 students. Some states had policies that allowed caseloads of 80. Some school-based SLPs reported caseloads as high as 100 (ASHA, 2002). Results of a study conducted by Blood, Swavely Ridenour, Thomas, and Qualls (2002) revealed that caseload size had a significant impact on job satisfaction, with professionals with lower caseloads reporting greater job satisfaction.

Caseload and Service Quality: Specific Effects

The ASHA (2002) examined the research related to caseload size in schools. The literature showed that large caseloads negatively affected speech-language services in five major ways: (1) by limiting service delivery options; (2) by roadblocking important professional activities necessary to meet the individual needs of students; (3) by impeding students' ability to make progress on individualized education program (IEP) goals; (4) by leading to burnout and attrition of school-based SLPs; and (5) by inhibiting compliance with federal mandates of providing free and appropriate services in the **least restrictive environment**. These negative effects are discussed next.

Limitation of Service Delivery Options

Despite the focus of IDEA '97 on collaboration and evidence that collaboration and consultation enhance inclusive practices, most school-based SLP services continued to be delivered through a pull-out model. SLPs from across the nation reported spending an average of 23 hours per week providing services using a pull-out model and serving students in groups rather than individually. Only two hours per week were devoted to consultation and collaboration, and classroom-based or curriculum-based services averaged only 1 hour per week. This limited involvement in collaboration, consultation, and classroom-based services appeared to be due in large part to the major challenges identified by school-based SLPs: high caseload sizes; lack of time for planning; collaborating and meeting with teachers; and burdensome amounts of paperwork (ASHA, 2001a, 2001b; Chiang & Rylance, 2000).

The ASHA **National Outcomes Measurement System** (NOMS) data confirmed that the vast majority of students (up to 92%) received speech-language intervention in pull-out groups. Two thirds of students were seen for services two times per week, and greater than 75% of those sessions ranged from 21 to 30 minutes in length (ASHA, 2000c). Data from the 1995 AHSA Schools Survey (Peters-Johnson, 1996, 1998) indicated almost no change in the service delivery options used by school-based SLPs in a decade. Paralleling the 2000 survey data, the pull-out group intervention model was the most common service delivery model in 1995 (total 86% of the time, 51% in group sessions, and 35% in individual sessions). The NOMS data report revealed that caseload size appeared to play a significant role in the way speech-language services were delivered (ASHA, 2000c; Karr & Schooling, 2001; Whitmire, Karr, & Mullen, 2000). Analyses indicated that increased caseload size resulted in a shift from individual to group services, as well as an increase in the number of students per group:

■ 31% of SLPs with caseloads greater than 60 students reported groups of 5 or more.
■ 6% of SLPs with caseloads of 40 or less reported treatment groups of five or more.
■ SLPS with caseloads of less than 40 children were more likely to provide individual services.
■ SLPs with caseloads less than 40 were more likely to use other service delivery models (classroom-based, collaborative

consultation, and so on) to treat their students.

These data suggested that a wider range of service delivery options would be available to a student if that student's SLP had a caseload of fewer than 40 students.

The ASHA Schools Survey (ASHA, 2004) revealed that more individual sessions were used in day or residential and preschools. In these settings, more than half of the population demonstrated severe or profound disabilities. More group sessions were used in elementary, secondary, and combined schools. Use of group sessions, however, did not necessarily yield lighter **workloads**. "Indeed, with the new and increased paperwork demands mandated by IDEA '97, the recent move for schools to bill other agencies, and an increase in the number of children with severe involved disabilities, a caseload of 40 strains even a dedicated professional" (Chiang & Rylance, 2000, p. 36).

These findings led Chiang and Rylance (2000) to make four major recommendations. First, the IEP and the needs of the student must be given priority. Second, caseloads should be of a size to allow SLPs to provide intervention services, collaborate and coteach, and complete the necessary paperwork in working hours. Third, caseloads composed of students with communication disorders should not exceed 40 under any circumstances. Fourth, caseloads containing students with severe and complex disabilities (e.g., autism, cognitive impairments, fetal alcohol syndrome, severe developmental delays) require substantial reduction to ensure provision of appropriate services.

Roadblock to Professional Activities to Meet Student Needs

Student communication outcomes appear to be strongly influenced by caseload size (ASHA, 2000b, 2001b). ASHA NOMS data show the following:

■ In comparing the proportion of students in grades kindergarten through sixth grade who made at least one level of progress on articulation goals, 87% of students on caseloads of less than 40 made measurable progress on their IEP goals. Only 63% of students on caseloads of 60 or more, however, made progress on the IEP goals.

■ An interaction existed between an SLP's caseload size and the teachers' perceptions regarding whether speech-language intervention improved students' reading comprehension and written language skills (Karr & Schooling, 2001). For students receiving remediation from SLPs with caseloads fewer than 40, 90% of general education teachers believed that these students demonstrated improved reading skills that were related to the services the SLP had provided. When the caseload size increased to 70, only 60% of the teachers felt that speech-language pathology services made a difference in students' reading abilities.

■ A shift from individual to group intervention made a difference in student outcomes (Karr & Schooling, 2001). Students were more likely to make measurable progress in speech sound production skills when they received individual treatment as opposed to group treatment.

■ A similar pattern was found for preschool children (ASHA, 2001c): 78% of children who received individual intervention services made progress toward improving their articulation, compared with 57% who received group intervention services.

Negative Impact on Students' Progress

When faced with high caseloads, SLPs tend to provide services in groups. Evidence-based practice data have shown that providing services in groups may not be the appropriate solution. Student progress often depends on the size of the group and the focus of the intervention program.

■ NOMS data (ASHA, 2001b) suggested that group intervention services were effective for preschool children with goals in the area of spoken language comprehension. Group size was one factor that appeared to affect students' verbal communication in ways that might in turn promote language development.

■ Lowenthal (1981) studied the effect of small-group instruction in comparison with large-group instruction as an approach to improving the oral language of preschoolers with delayed language. Students were assigned to control (large) or experimental (small) groups. Students in small groups of 3 made significantly greater gains in **receptive vocabulary**, **auditory comprehension**, and verbal ability than those noted for students in large groups of 10 children.

■ McCabe, Jenkins, Mills, Dale, Cole, and Pepler (1996) found differences between playgroup sizes of two and four in the amount of **expressive language** that students with disabilities used with peers. Students with disabilities used significantly more **utterances** per minute when playing in groups of two, but when placed in groups of four, they produced fewer utterances, although they used a larger number of different words.

■ Increased practice with talking appeared to facilitate vocabulary growth and complex sentence production in students with disabilities (Hart & Risley, 1980). When placed in larger groups, however, young students with communication disabilities talked approximately half as much as their typically developing peers and were much less responsive to inquiries from teachers and peers (Warren & Rogers-Warren, 1982).

These results suggested that students with the most severe language disabilities tend not to engage in the practice they need for language development (i.e., increased talking time). Therefore, providing speech-language intervention services in smaller groups (with a student-to-staff ratio of 3:1

or less) may provide students with more opportunities for conversational participation and verbal communication. Use of smaller student-to-staff ratios may maximize talking practice and lead to improved communication outcomes for students with speech-language disabilities.

Burnout and Attrition of School-Based Speech-Language Pathologists

The trend of increasing **caseload** and the increased responsibilities of teachers appear to be important factors contributing to high rates of teacher attrition in the field of special education, including speech-language pathology. If the current attrition rates continue, it has been predicted that some districts may not be able to meet the federal requirements of IDEA '04 to provide a free and appropriate public education for all students with disabilities (Wisniewski & Gargiulo, 1997). For speech-language pathology, greater than 50% of respondents to the 2000 ASHA Schools Survey reported a shortage of qualified SLPs in their school district (ASHA, 2000d). The effects of this shortage on service delivery, as indicated by the respondents, included the following:

- Increased caseload (80%)
- Decreased opportunities for individual services (62%)
- Decreased quality of service (58%)

Findings on school SLP shortages from 1995 were remarkably similar to those in current research. ASHA survey data reported by Peters-Johnson (1996, 1998) indicated that 60% of respondents reported SLP shortages in their districts. Respondents who reported shortages felt that the major impacts on the shortages of service delivery were increased caseload and decreased quality of service. For a majority of respondents seen in the ASHA 2000 schools survey on SLPs' working conditions, their greatest challenges were burdensome paperwork (88%), lack of time for planning, collaboration, and meeting with teachers (81%), and high caseload (60%). These results were similar to those from the 1995 ASHA schools survey (Peters-Johnson, 1996, 1998), when most respondents indicated that the greatest challenges in their jobs were large caseloads, paperwork, and time limitations.

During the 1990s, state education agencies were beginning to examine the impact of high caseloads on SLP services for students in schools. There appeared to be a strong relationship between working conditions and SLP shortages. For example, the Ohio Legislature (Ohio Legislative Office of Education Oversight, 1999) determined that schools had difficulty finding SLPs primarily because the working conditions in schools were less favorable than in most health care settings. Specifically, this study indicated that the public school work environment often included larger caseloads; in schools, SLPs served over 50 students in groups, whereas in health care, they served between 16 and 30 clients in one-on-one sessions. School SLPs also reported that paperwork was particularly excessive for school districts seeking reimbursement from Medicaid for services. Data from this study also confirmed results from the 2000 ASHA survey on how SLP shortages affected students. When shortages occurred, approximately 60% of SLPs and school administrators surveyed in Ohio reported that frequency of sessions were reduced; 57% reported that the duration of sessions was reduced; 30% reported that students went without services; and 20% stated that students received services from noncertified staff. An alarming finding reported by 87% of respondents was that students were affected by SLP shortages.

Several studies have looked specifically at job satisfaction in school SLPs (Banks & Necco, 1990; Chiang & Rylance, 2000; Goldberg, 1993; Miller & Potter, 1982; Pezzei & Oratio, 1991). These studies have consistently shown that public school SLPs with large caseloads, increased paperwork, and funding cuts were particularly susceptible to burnout. As the volume of workload or caseload increased, the degree of job burnout increased. These appeared to be the same factors that were reported to contribute to personnel shortages of SLPs in schools (e.g., Ohio Legislative Office of Education Oversight, 1999). Many special educators have reported that increases in caseloads correspond with simultaneous increases in meetings and paperwork demands (Russ, Chiang, Rylance, & Bongers, 2001). Each student added to the caseload increases the time needed not only for evaluation, diagnosis, and service but also for paperwork, multidisciplinary conferences, parent and teacher contact, and many other responsibilities. Multiplying the number of students on the SLP caseload by the number of forms that must be completed per student and the number of meetings that must be attended provided an initial indication of the time implications of this factor (ASHA, 2003).

Chiang and Rylance (2000) researched school SLPs' perceptions of working conditions. With specific regard to caseloads, 75% reported that caseload affected job satisfaction; 81% indicated that caseload affected their job effectiveness; 83% reported that high caseload negatively affected the type of intervention services used; and 83% reported that caseload affected their ability to engage in collaboration with other teachers. Chiang and Rylance concluded that the responses of the SLPs surveyed clearly pointed to professional responsibilities' being met minimally. Open-ended responses indicated that time pressures were prevalent and that it was not possible to provide appropriate intervention for a large caseload while doing paperwork, conducting necessary phone calls, and attending meetings. The ASHA Schools Survey (ASHA, 2004) revealed that the greatest impact of NCLB has been increased paperwork and increased time in prereferral activities.

Inhibition of Compliance with IDEA '04 and the Mandate for Free Appropriate Public Education

IDEA '04 (PL 94-142) (U.S. Congress, 1997; U.S. Dept. of Education, 2000) ensured provision of the following for students with disabilities:

- A **free and appropriate public education** (FAPE)
- Education in the least restrictive environment possible
- A continuum of service options in placements designed to meet the individual needs of each student

- Access to and a connection with the general education curriculum
- A collaborative approach involving various education professionals
- Enhanced parent involvement

Professional and special education groups have reinforced the intent of the federal mandates with numerous position statements advocating that each student with a disability should be provided with a continuum of service options that will guarantee a free, appropriate public education based on that student's specific needs. Both the ASHA (1996) and the National Joint Committee on Learning Disabilities (1993) supported the use of a continuum of services and rejected the arbitrary placement of all students in any one setting. These groups have recommended the use of a variety of models through which inclusive practices can be provided, including direct (pull-out) programs, classroom-based service delivery, and consultative interventions. These models should be seen as flexible options that may change according to student needs. The SLP, in collaboration with parents, the student, teachers, support personnel, and administrators, is in the ideal position to decide the model or combination of models that best serves each student's communication needs. Although speech-language caseloads have remained essentially unchanged over the past decade (ASHA, 2000d; Peters-Johnson, 1992), the role of the school-based SLP has changed dramatically (ASHA, 1991, 1999, 2001b; Beck & Dennis, 1997; Cirrin & Penner, 1995; Eger, 1992; Ehren, 2000; Elksnin & Capilouto, 1994; Prelock, 2000).

Additional federal and state requirements to ensure increased student access to general education programs and curriculum, consideration of assistive technology, and billing government agencies and health insurance companies are just a few examples of mandated responsibilities that did not exist a decade ago. Similarly, increased workload responsibilities have been noted in such areas as communication with parents, general and special education teachers, and administrators; participation on teams; paperwork requirements; and supervising the work of paraprofessionals. As mentioned previously, the results of NCLB has been increased paperwork and increased time spent by SLPs with prereferral activities (ASHA, 2004). The standards of what constitute a "reasonable" caseload today are much different from those accepted 10 years ago. IDEA '04, in particular, has increased the responsibilities of the school-based SLP. With the IDEA '04 reauthorization, the following changes in the practice of most school-based SLPs are recognized:

- SLPs serve more children with complex communication disorders that require intensive, long-term interventions. Students with more severe disabilities may require greater use of individualized and smaller group models of service delivery as well as more frequent contact every week (U.S. Department of Education, 2000).
- SLPs serve more students who are medically fragile or who have multiple disabilities. The U.S. Department of Education (2000) reported that the most common service for children with two or more co-occurring disabilities was speech-language intervention services. In addition, students with co-occurring disabilities often received services from a variety of providers, resulting in a need for greater collaboration in planning and providing these services.
- SLPs provide services in the least restrictive environment and through the general education curriculum whenever possible and appropriate. This requirement means additional planning and collaboration time with other teachers and professionals.
- SLPs play important direct and indirect roles in facilitating literacy for children with and without communication disorders (ASHA, 2001b). The roles and responsibilities of SLPs with respect to reading and writing in children and adolescents have included prevention, identification, assessment, intervention, monitoring and follow-up evaluation.

School-based SLPs who were not aware of the research data discussed in this chapter built their weekly schedules solely on **direct services** (i.e., what is done with students), because they were focusing on the caseload. In the era of NCLB and IDEA '04, school-based SLPs must learn how to focus on workload. They must to learn how to build a schedule based not only on what they do with students but also on what they do for and on behalf of students. Large caseloads constrained the SLP's ability and capacity to engage in the expanded roles necessary to meet individual needs within diverse and complex student populations.

What Is Caseload?

As reported by the ASHA (2000a, 2000b, 2000c, 2000d, 2000e), *caseload* may not be limited to the number of students who have IEPs or **individualized family service plans** (IFSPs). In some school districts, the SLP's caseload also may include students who are enrolled in a response to intervention program and those who receive prereferral services. The caseload also may include students for whom the SLP serves as the **case manager**.

What Is Workload?

Caseload is one component of workload. However, *workload* goes beyond the focus of direct services provided to students and includes all of the professional activities for which an SLP is held responsible. By making the shift from caseload to workload, the school-based SLP must be able to focus on the individual needs of students, document the full range of his or her responsibilities in activities performed not only with but also for and on behalf of those students, and use that documentation in dialogue with her or his administration. Five major premises are embodied in the concept of workload:

- First, every student added to the caseload carries additional workload responsibilities. Each student added to the caseload increases the time needed not only for evaluation, diagnosis, direct services, and **indirect services** but also for mandated ongoing assessment, paperwork, conferencing, parent contacts, professional collaboration, and other related responsibilities such as supervising para-educators and providing technical support.

- Second, workload is affected by the severity of the disability of a student, as well as the frequency and duration of required services.
- Third, caseloads must be of a size that allows SLPs to carry out all mandated duties.
- Fourth, education agencies must implement a workload analysis approach so that SLPs may engage in the broad range of professional activities necessary to meet the individual needs of each student.
- Finally, use of a workload approach gives the SLP and administrators a common ground by which a caseload can be analyzed. The SLP is seen as a professional concerned about being in compliance with mandates and dedicated to meeting all of the needs of students.

The use of a workload approach to determine the number of students who can be adequately and appropriately served has been receiving serious attention from special education and other professionals, including those employed in state and local education agencies and school-based occupational and physical therapy programs (Hylton, 1987), clinical supervisors in university training programs (Johnson & Meline, 1997), school psychologists (Keith, 1992), child welfare workers (Stein, Callaghan, McGee, & Douglas, 1990; Mills & Ivery, 1991), and itinerant teachers of the vision-impaired (Olmstead, 1995). In a balanced workload approach designed to meet individual student needs, caseload is conceptualized as only one part of a school-based SLP's workload. The ASHA (2002) recommended that workload be viewed as consisting of four categories: (1) direct services; (2) indirect services that support educational services; (3) indirect services that support the least restrictive environment; and (4) activities that support compliance with laws.

Direct Services

Identification, evaluation, and direct intervention/instruction are the traditional hallmarks of school-based SLP services. Implementation of students' IEPs on an individual basis or in small groups and decisions regarding scheduling direct services are bound by factors such as length of the school day and specifications in students' IEPs.

Indirect Services That Support Educational Services

IDEA '04 strengthened the requirement for special education services to be provided in the least restrictive environment and to be aligned with the general education curriculum. Student-centered activities that support compliance with delivery of services in a least restrictive environment include classroom observations, teacher interviews, pre-referral interventions, curriculum considerations, and dynamic assessment.

Indirect Services That Support the Mandate of Least Restrictive Environment

Various activities performed by SLPs require the application of clinical skills outside of a direct service setting. For example, the design, maintenance, programming, and staff training for assistive technology and augmentative communication systems constitute clinical work that is required to support students. Other associated activities that involve student-centered planning and collaboration with other professionals outside of direct instruction or intervention with students include proactive behavior plans; prereferral consultation; curriculum and instructional modifications; service plan design; data collection and analysis; communication and planning with private, nonpublic school teachers and staff; and transition planning. Time must be scheduled weekly or monthly in order to complete these activities on behalf of students with communication disorders.

Activities That Support Compliance with Laws

Speech-language service in schools is a compliance-driven industry. Accountability is required in the form of student evaluation reports, the written IEP for each student receiving special education, progress reports, daily charts, third party billing statements, funding reports, and student count reports. In addition, as a member of the school community, the SLP may participate in activities such as staff meetings, faculty meetings, assigned school duty, professional development, campus or district committees, curriculum committees, and other professional activities. By involvement in such activities, the SLP interfaces with other educators who are partners in the education of all students. Policies and procedures

that affect all students, in academic as well as unstructured school environments, may be influenced. Table 2–1 provides an example of workload activities categorized into four areas. By examining these four areas, SLPs may analyze the "time pie" based not only on what must be done with students, but also what must be done for and on behalf of students.

Considerations Regarding Options for Unmet Needs

Although the main responsibilities of school-based SLPs will be similar across settings, individual SLPs, school districts, and schools must establish their own priorities. Meeting individual student

Table 2–1. Categories of Activities for the School-Based Speech-Language Pathologist

Curriculum-Related Activities	Administrative/ Management Tasks	Direct Intervention	Associated Student-Centered Activities
Curriculum considerations	Writing IEPs with team	Identification	Designing AAC tools
Consultation with teachers	Writing student evaluation reports	Assessment	Environmental modifications
Designing modifications		Evaluation	
Classroom observations	Writing daily logs	Reevaluation	Teacher and staff training
Designing adaptations	Writing student progress reports	Intervention	Referral to other agencies
Dynamic assessment		Counseling	Interagency communications
Responsiveness to intervention programs	Documenting procedural safeguards	IEP activities	Transition planning
Prereferral consultation	Third party billing		Connecting academic standards to IEP goals
Screening	Professional development		
Faculty/staff meetings	Supervision		Collecting data
Prevention	Travel time		Implementing IEP activities
IEP activities	School improvement teams		
	Planning time		
	School duties and committees		
	Professional associations		

AAC = adaptive-augmentative communication; IEP = individualized education program.

needs is always the key focus of activities consistent with the requirements of IDEA '04. Using a balanced workload methodology to determine the importance of all required activities allows the SLP to determine how time and energies are best spent. Construction of the workload (see balanced workload matrix below) to which activities have been assigned allows the objective consideration of what the workload looks like, which activities are consuming the time of the SLP, and how activities can be balanced to meet students' individual needs. Systematic and graphical representation of the responsibilities of the SLP allows administrative analysis as well. Administrators of programs are responsible for ensuring that a school district is in compliance with both state and federal legal mandates. Viewing the activities and assigning time commitments associated with the activities allow both the SLP and the program administrator to determine whether adjustment is necessary to ensure increased student achievement, and which activities need to be reprioritized for students to meet IEP and IFSP goals.

The conceptual shift from caseload to the calculation of workload requires a systems change. SLPs and school administrators must commit time and effort to identify the steps needed to effect this change and implement a strategy that will ensure appropriate speech-language services for children. Thoughtful consideration must be given to the key elements of such a systems change. The inclusion of a variety of persons, such as teachers, administrators, and parents, in the planning and implementation will ensure a higher degree of success. This change will result in the assignment of new responsibilities, the addition of professional or support staff, or the realignment of staffing patterns.

Twelve Steps to a Workload Analysis

The following strategies are intended to help SLPs and administrators chart a course for analysis of workload. The 12 steps delineated here address self-assessment, planning, monitoring, and full implementation.

Step 1

Look at required workload activities, instead of focusing exclusively on caseload. To implement the changes discussed here, it will be critical to change the paradigm with which most SLPs have become familiar. This conceptual shift from the discussion of *caseload* to *workload* is perhaps the most important, yet most difficult, step toward success. Most people enter the field of speech-language pathology with a deep desire to work with students, and direct intervention often becomes the singular focus of the professional's workload. Examination of a typical school-based SLP's weekly schedule will show that most of the time slots are filled with the names of students. SLPs need to learn how to stop scheduling just students and how to start scheduling workload responsibilities. As reported by Sally Disney, an SLP practicing in Ohio, "Our office has always told our SLPs to relate all aspects of their schedule in a workload analysis to specific students whenever possible rather than to just write a word like planning, which can be misunderstood. It helps administrators relate to time-intense students in a realistic way" (S. Disney, personal communication, November 20, 2004). Making the conceptual shift from caseload to workload may pose a challenge that requires a **metacognitive** process and an attitude adjustment. It is essential to collaborate with administrators and policymakers starting with step one and continuing through the entire process. Workload analysis outcomes will only be as effective as the amount of support given from the policymakers, administrators, and all parties involved in the process.

Step 2

Analyze the current work week. Once the conceptual shift has been made, it is important to look at the job responsibilities from this new perspective. A balanced workload will certainly include direct instruction, interventions using clinical skills and curriculum-related activities (e.g., identification, evaluation, reevaluation, remediation, interventions, counseling, the implementation of IEPs and IFSPs). Also critical to a balanced workload will be the administrative and management tasks, general curriculum-related activities, and associated student-centered activities that must be acknowledged, analyzed, and implemented. Each SLP should ask, "Where am I spending my time? Where *should* I be spending my time?" In describing mandated workload activities, it is essential to consider state and federal legal requirements.

Step 3

Once the workload has been identified and clearly defined, and mandates have been documented using legal references, determine whether there is a match or a mismatch between time and workload. If there is a mismatch, it is essential to doc-

ument concerns and provide concrete examples of undesirable outcomes when specific aspects of the workload are not honored. The examples should be referenced to the relevant legal mandates. Begin by filling slots in the weekly or monthly schedule with time needed for the "fixed" tasks " such as Administrative/Management Tasks, in Table 2–1. It may be helpful to consider the average number of hours per week or month that is taken up by these administrative activities. Factors to consider include contracted time for planning, contracted time for lunch, travel between schools, case management duties, assessment time, evaluation time, due process documentation, third party billing, and duty assignments (e.g., lunch duty, hall duty, bus duty). A typical schedule might look like the one shown in Figure 2–1.

Time	Monday	Tuesday	Wednesday	Thursday	Friday
7:45–8:00	Hall duty	Hall duty	Hall duty	Hall duty	Hall duty
8:00–8:40	Prereferral team	Intervention	Observations	Intervention	Observations
8:40–9:20	Preparation	Communications	Preparation	Intervention	Preparation
9:20–10:00	Intervention	Preparation	Intervention	Preparation	Intervention
10:00–10:40	Intervention	Intervention	Intervention	Intervention	Intervention
10:40–11:20	Intervention	Intervention	Intervention	Intervention	Intervention
11:20–12:00	Travel	Travel	Travel	Travel	Travel
12:00–12:30	Lunch	Lunch	Lunch	Lunch	Lunch
12:30–1:10	Intervention	Intervention	Intervention	Intervention	Intervention
1:10–1:50	Intervention	Intervention	Intervention	Intervention	Intervention
1:50–2:30	Assessment	Intervention	Assessment	Intervention	Assessment
2:30–3:10	Consultation	Assessment	Consultation	Assessment	Consultation
3:10–3:30	Logs/billing	Logs/billing	Logs/billing	Logs/billing	Logs/billing
3:30–4:00	IEP meetings	Committee meetings	IEP meetings	Faculty meetings	AAC designs

Figure 2–1. Typical hourly/weekly schedule for a school-based speech-language pathologist. AAC, adaptive-augmentative communication.

Step 4

Determine the activities necessary to provide appropriate intervention services in accord with the intent of IDEA '04 for each student on the caseload. In effect, this step can be conceptualized as an analysis of each student's needs. It may be helpful to use the balanced workload matrix (ASHA, 2002) for this step. Slots in the SLP's weekly or monthly schedule are likely be filled by tasks from student-centered services depending on the needs of each student. Then the IEP team should discuss how to best facilitate the student's progress on functional communication abilities. As the team explores student service options, consideration must be given to service parameters as they relate to IDEA '04 mandates, best practices in school speech-language pathology, and the evidence-based research reviewed in this chapter. Factors to consider include the following:

■ The most appropriate service delivery model
■ Resources to facilitate a continuum of service delivery options
■ Activities spent on behalf of the student; document these on the student support services page of the IEP
■ Need for classroom consultation
■ Time needed to program any adaptive-augmentative communication (AAC) devices
■ Type and severity of the student's disability
■ The age of the student
■ The grade of the student
■ The communication goals that the SLP is the only professional uniquely trained to address
■ The natural communication supports available in the student's environment
■ Opportunities to interface the student's goals with the general education curriculum
■ Amount and frequency of service required

Step 5

Start filling available slots with necessary student services. Some considerations in this aspect of preparation for workload analysis follow:

■ It is critical to have data-based and supportable time estimates for all activities in the workload.
■ Administrators and principals must be aware that every single activity and task performed to meet the intent of IDEA '04 and other state and local requirements takes time out of the workday, which adds up over the course of a week.
■ When a student is added to the caseload, additional time for all of the support activities must be accounted for (factor in all relevant activities from the four categories in Table 2–1).
■ Slots may also be filled according to state and local procedures, which will vary by district and by school. For example, some districts hold IEP meetings during the general education teacher's preparation period. This may take up a direct intervention service slot during the precious hours of the school day.

Step 6

Strive for balance among four categories in Table 2–1, in accordance with caseload and the needs of individual students. Task balance may look different at different times of the school year depending on semester or seasonal variations in the tasks and responsibilities necessary to support students on the speech-language caseload and whether cyclic or block scheduling is used. Balance tasks across categories for each student.

Step 7

Identify when all of the time slots are filled. When all available slots are filled, caseload maximum has been reached for this particular set of circumstances (school, caseload, severity, and so on), and the intent of IDEA '04 has been fulfilled. When the workload responsibilities do not fit into the time slots available, the SLP and the school district must explore possible options for change. The following five questions can be used to guide this process:

- What is the current workload problem?
- What effect is the problem having on students?
- What can be done?
- Who can help?
- What is a reasonable plan of action?

Step 8

Identify the problem. When the problem of workload management has been clearly identified, documented, and described in student-centered terms, explore all possible solutions. Each SLP must design a solution, tailored to his or her individual situation, that addresses the specific workload components. It is wise to develop a number of possible options or initiatives (e.g., Plan A, Plan B, and Plan C) so that success does not hinge on a single initiative. Flexibility becomes an important consideration at this step.

Step 9

Identify the policy makers who could support the desired change. When Plans A, B, and C have been clearly defined, take time to develop a brief, written summary of the problems, the initiatives already taken that have helped relieve the problems, and the additional initiatives that must be taken to achieve success. Make appointments with each policy maker responsible for some aspect of change (e.g., team leader, principal, director of special education, superintendent). Provide each policy maker with the same summary so that each person has identical information from which to make decisions. Determine which option (A, B, or C) appears to be most

acceptable among the policy makers. Important to this step is the determination of which policy makers will offer the most support when the advocacy step is begun.

Step 10

Develop an advocacy plan of action. Once the options have been explored and new initiatives developed, it is important to develop a written plan of action. This plan will provide the framework for a process to calculate workload activities and that ensure student success.

Step 11

Pilot the new plan for one year through a collaborative team effort. It is advisable to identify one or more pilot sites to implement the plan for one school year. In large systems, it may be appropriate to have numerous pilots to account for all of the features of the action plan. In selecting the pilot site(s), it is important to identify persons who voice support for the change and commitment to success. Data from the pilot will become critical in making adjustments to the plan. At the completion of the pilot year, the process can be refined by making such adjustments, and the workload approach can be implemented districtwide. It is recommended to include the full staff of SLPs in the discussion and implementation of adjustments to the plan. This helps to ensure a sense of ownership and commitment to districtwide implementation.

Step 12

Stay flexible. Make additions, deletions, corrections, and modifications to the action plan. Even the most carefully crafted plans can benefit from some type of modification, based on trial, input, and assessment. The input acquired from the self-monitoring activity and the critique from other professionals should yield recommendations for adjustment. It is important to consider these additions, deletions, corrections, and modifications to the pilot in an effort to fine-tune the process of determining workload.

Conduct self-monitoring at several points during the pilot year. Implementation during the pilot year must include an opportunity to check the progress of change. A schedule should be developed to identify two or three opportunities throughout the pilot year to look closely at the key strategies defined in the action plan. The self-monitoring activity should be conducted by the same team of people who developed the action plan, with input provided by any stakeholders who shared some involvement with the implementation of the pilot. The key points of the action plan should be monitored using factual data, with careful attention to eliminate bias or opinion.

Solicit input from others (parents, professionals, students, and administrators). Valuable information will be collected in the self-monitoring activity, but it is important to solicit input from a wider circle of people who are affected by the change. Interviews, questionnaires, and written input constitute a variety of means for collecting this critique. As with any constructive criticism, it is important to acknowledge this input and make appropriate changes if necessary. Keep in mind that input from different groups of people may appear to be contradictory. In such instances, it is the responsibility of the decision makers to review the input and determine what action should be taken.

Some Workload Solutions

The workload analysis approach to caseload standards in schools can be time consuming and may appear to be a daunting task for the professional who already feels overloaded. Use of the workload analysis approach, however, has made a significant difference for professionals who have invested their time in its application. The ASHA Schools Survey (ASHA, 2004) revealed that 61% of the survey respondents found the workload analysis approach to be helpful in their work settings.

All of the workload solutions offered in this section are currently being used by SLPs in public schools today. Many of these strategies have been used successfully for several years. The workload solutions are categorized into service delivery options, administrative options, and contract options. Initiating any of these workload solutions will require a cooperative effort among teachers, administrators, parents, and other professionals.

Service Delivery Options

Changing the way service is delivered to students may result in a lighter workload even though the caseload number remains the same. A variety of service delivery options have been developed by school-based SLPs across the United States. The service delivery options described here have been successfully implemented. Other modes of service delivery may be developed in accordance with the needs of the students on the caseload, the roles and responsibilities of the SLP, the needs of the general education teachers, the level of administrative support, the needs of the school district, and input from parents, caregivers, and legal guardians.

Supportive Teaching

In the **supportive teaching** service delivery model, the SLP teaches information related to the curriculum while incorporating IEP goals into the lesson. Rather than holding three pull-out sessions per week, the SLP does a preteaching session in the pull-out room. The second session is conducted in a classroom as a group lesson. The classroom teacher also is in the room and either observes or monitors student performance. The third session is again held in the pull-out room for post-lesson clarification or test adaptations. The SLP and the classroom teacher share responsibility for planning the program, monitoring the progress of students, dealing with behavioral issues, and making decisions about modifying the program. The SLP uses this model in kindergarten through fifth grade. Communications with each classroom teacher is conducted via a monthly questionnaire that goes back and forth between mailboxes. Face-to-face meetings are conducted twice a month with each group of grade-level teachers. By shifting to this model, the SLP now has more time to devote to workload issues, rather than spending all available time providing direct caseload sessions.

Complementary Teaching

In the **complementary teaching** service delivery model, the SLP provides services in the classroom setting. The classroom teacher presents most of the content of the lesson, and the SLP focuses on related skills such as learning science vocabulary, sequencing the steps of an assignment, or paraphrasing the main ideas of an assignment. Both partners teach in the classroom from their own areas of expertise. They share responsibilities for planning the program, teaching the lessons, monitoring the progress of the students, and making decisions about modifying the program. The SLP and the classroom teacher address the goals on the IEPs for the children in the classroom. Some students still require services provided in a pull-out program. By shifting to a complementary teaching model, the SLP has been able to free up time for workload issues, rather than spending all her time doing direct caseload sessions. The SLP also is able to cut his or her conference time with teachers because the teachers are able to directly observe specific teaching techniques used with students in the classroom.

Consultation

In the **consultation/consultative intervention** service delivery model, the SLP works outside the classroom to analyze, adapt, modify, or create appropriate instructional materials. The adapted materials may be for one child, for several children, or for an entire classroom. The SLP does not teach in the classroom but does do classroom observations. The students come to the speech-language room for one period per day for skill support or test adaptations. Working together, the SLP and the teacher plan, monitor, and make decisions about materials. By shifting to a resource

management model, the SLP now has more time to spend on workload issues.

Team Teaching

In the **team teaching** model, the SLP, the learning disabilities teacher, the behavioral disabilities teacher, the cognitive disabilities teacher, and the general education classroom teacher all work together to address the IEP goals for all children. One special educator serves as a resource person for each grade level in grades 5 through 8. The adolescents come to the speech-language room, by grade level, for one period per day. The SLP assigns grades on their report cards. At the middle school and high school levels, the services may be presented as a course for credit if curriculum-based goals are met. Shifting to this model may allow the SLP to free up to three class periods per day to deal with workload issues.

The team teaching model also is applicable at the preschool level. Patricia Wildgen, an SLP practicing in Ohio, used a team teaching model, when she was the only SLP, to help begin the Integrated Preschool Project in an Akron City School. Children with special needs were integrated into Head Start classrooms with a team teaching approach. A pull-out model for delivery of speech-language services was used only 2% of the time. The rest of the time was spent providing services from various educators and other professionals who made up a core team.

Resource Room

In the **resource room** model, the SLP, learning disabilities teacher, the behavioral disabilities teacher, and the cognitive disabilities teacher provide support for communication skills, basic skills, social skills, and study skills. Adolescents come to a resource room for one or two periods per day instead of going to a study hall. The special educators integrate the IEP goals into curriculum-based strategies and support as the students complete assignments. At the middle school and high school levels, the services may be presented as a course taken for credit if curriculum-based goals are met.

Diagnostic Speech-Language Pathology Services

The school may employ an SLP who serves as a **diagnostician**. The diagnostic SLP attends all IEP meetings, completes all legal paperwork, meets with parents, and helps develop the IEPs. This SLP may or may not provide direct services to other students, depending on the workload involved in the diagnostic activities.

Speech Club

In the **speech club** model, the SLP is assigned to lunchroom duty Mondays through Thursdays. The SLP uses this time to monitor students on the caseload who are in carryover phases of their program. Each student invites a classmate to join her or him for lunch at the speech club table. The SLP monitors the communication skills of the students in this unstructured setting. The SLP's half-hour, duty-free lunch break is scheduled for a different time of the day, to allow more time during the day for workload issues.

Teaming for Reading Instruction

In the **teaming for reading** model, an SLP teams up with five other team members: a reading specialist, a learning disabilities teacher, an occupational therapist, an occupational therapist assistant, and an educational assistant. The team members work together to teach reading instruction to all of the children in general education and special education.

The program operates Monday through Thursday. All children in first grade are given 30 minutes of the reading curriculum 4 days per week. This is accompanied by 25 minutes of language comprehension instruction 4 days per week and 25 minutes of fine motor instruction once per week. This program results in a coordinated language and reading program for all children. It includes sequential and multisensory phonics instruction, phonological awareness, story grammar, vocabulary development, comprehension development, reasoning skills development, letter formation, and fine motor skills development.

Each educator involved in the program teaches from his or her strength. The SLP focuses on phonological awareness, story grammar, vocabulary building, comprehension, and reasoning skill development. The occupational therapist and the educational assistant focus on letter formation and fine motor skill development. The reading specialist and the learning disabilities teacher focus on the sequential, multisensory phonics instruction. By using this inclusive practice approach, the SLP has more time to devote to workload aspects of his or her position, rather than just dealing with caseloads. "Integrated phonological awareness intervention may be an efficient method to improve phonological awareness, speech production, and reading development of children with SLI" (Gillon, 2000, p. 126).

Administrative Options

Some school districts may opt to use a districtwide workload policy, rather than a variety of workload solutions that vary from school to school. Specific administrative solutions that have worked for school-based SLPs across the nation are presented next.

Early Release Day

The school district designates one day each week as an "early release day" or a "late start day." The students are dismissed an hour early or arrive an hour later than usual. General education teachers and special education teachers work together on curriculum modifications. SLPs also may use this time for work-related activities.

Program Support Teachers

School districts may use federal dollars to fund **program support teachers** (PSTs) who are fully certified SLPs. PSTs can assume some of the workload responsibilities for the district SLPs. PSTs may assist with evaluation, programming, and placement of students with disabilities; serve on IEP teams; assist in planning intervention strategies; coordinate communications among schools and other agencies; communicate with parents; provide resources and information; assist in procurement of appropriate materials and equipment; and assist in planning intervention strategies for specific students. Thus, PSTs relieve some of the workload responsibilities that otherwise would fall on the shoulders of the SLP.

Diversified Roles

In the **diversified roles** approach, two (or more) SLPs may be assigned to each school. One SLP deals with all of the students on the caseload with whom inclusive practices must be used. The other SLP deals with all of the students who require pull-out services. This approach allows both SLPs to spend more time on workload-related issues. Gwen Robl, an SLP practicing in Wenaukee, Wisconsin, has reported success with use of a diversified roles approach even when another SLP was not available. In her success story, she shared workload with another special educator who was certified in the area of learning disabilities. Both professionals served different children with similar needs in the same classrooms. The learning disabilities specialist wrote the test modifications, and then Robl created the study guide. With collaborative discussion, the particular needs of the students on the SLP's caseload and the needs of the students on the learning disabilities specialist's caseload were met through a joint effort. Robl also reported using a diversified roles approach with other general educators and special educators. Each professional contributed to the creation of a shared files system. The shared files were housed on a computer drive and consisted of curriculum adaptations, test adaptations, vocabulary lists, and modified worksheets for each grade-level curriculum and related activities. For example, Robl could go to a file for a sixth grade science unit and find materials prepared by various general education and special education teachers. She could find several versions of a specific unit test and also find several versions of accommodated tests. The shared file system grew over several years. Everyone involved agreed that it was usually easier to start with something other than the blank page when modifying materials to meet the specific needs of each individual (G. Robl, personal communication, August 15, 2005).

Contract Options

In some school districts, neither service delivery options nor administrative options can be used because of the unique circumstances of the local school districts. In such cases, contract options have been explored and developed. Examples of successful contract options that have been used across the nation are presented next.

Workload Week

For the **workload week** option, language is written into the teacher contract that recognizes all of the roles and responsibilities of the SLP. IEPs may be written to specify minutes per month, rather than minutes per week, or the number of minutes per week for each task is clearly defined in the IEP. An example of IEP wording specifying minutes per week follows:

> *Week 1*: 30 min. = direct individual intervention 3 times per week; 20 min. = consultation with autism specialist; 10 min. = writing in notebook for parents

> *Week 2*: 30 min. = direct individual intervention 2 times per week; 30 min. = direct group intervention; 20 min. = consultation with autism specialist; 10 min. = writing in notebook for parents

> *Week 3*: 30 min. = direct individual intervention; 30 min. = direct group intervention 2 times per week; 20 min. = consultation with autism specialist; 10 min. = writing in notebook for parents

> *Week 4*: 0 min. = direct individual intervention; 0 min. = direct group intervention; 30 min. = classroom observation 3 times per week; 30 min. = speech club; 30 min. = team meeting; 30 min. = observation on the playground

The last full week of each month is devoted to workload-related activities. The SLP does not see students for direct services during this week unless it is for assessment and evaluation purposes. Smaller school districts do the same thing but use a 6-week rotation schedule, rather than a monthly rotation. Another option would be to designate one day or one-half day per week for workload-related activities.

Weighted Formula

A **weighted formula** can be used to determine caseload sizes. The caseload numbers take into account time to do the following workload activities: professional collaboration, parent contacts, inservice training, service delivery options, supervision and communication with support staff, travel time, schedule issues, planning time, service on building assistance teams, committee work, duties (e.g., hallways, bus, playground, lunchroom), development of alternate assessments, and development of alternative curricula and materials.

Compensation Language

Compensation language can be written into the master contract for psychologists, diagnosticians, and SLPs. SLPs are assigned caseloads no larger than a district-determined maximum number without additional compensation. In the event that an SLP is assigned a caseload that exceeds the maximum number per a monthly caseload report, that SLP receives compensation in the amount of 3% of his or her salary per student. Such compensation is paid in biweekly units on a quarterly basis until such time as the child is dismissed through the IEP process or until the date the child leaves the school. SLPs also are provided one-half day per week to deal with other workload activities. In appropriate cases, overload assignments may result in reduction of preparation time. Choosing between compensation and assistance by additional staff is at the school district's discretion.

Success Story: A Workload Analysis Approach Applied to a Weighting System

Heidi Notbohm, an SLP practicing in Middleton, Wisconsin, is a seasoned professional with more than 25 years of public school experience. Her experience and wisdom told her that, if she wanted to help her school district make the conceptual shift from caseload to workload, she would have to work within the existing system. Nothom's employer, the Middleton/Cross Plains Area School District (MCPASD), used a weighted workload formula for programs that serve students with cognitive disabilities, learning disabilities, and behavioral disabilities, but no similar formula was in use for speech-language programs.

Notbohm and some of her colleagues attended the presentation on "A Workload Analysis Approach to Caseload Standards in Schools" at the 2003 ASHA Convention. This motivated Notbohm to form an ad hoc committee within the group of SLPs employed in the school district. The ad hoc committee worked diligently during the 2003–2004 academic year; provided monthly progress reports to all district SLPs; and sought their input and feedback every step of the way. As a result of feedback from the larger group, the committee learned that workload activities differed at the elementary and the secondary levels. As a result, weighting categories were defined differently for the two levels.

When the conceptual framework was built, Notbohm and her committee members met with Erin Kuehn, the MCPASD Director of Student Services, and Sherri Cyra, an elementary school principal in the school system. Cyra was a strong supporter of the workload-weighted formula. She had recently changed her principalship from one elementary school to another and could see a dramatic difference in workload because of the differences in the student populations between the two schools. Cyra agreed to be the information liaison to all of the other principals in the school district. On receiving input from the principals and Erin Kuehn, Director of Student Services, additional modifications were made to the weighted workload formula. The final draft was distributed to all of the SLPs in the school district. Each SLP was asked to apply the weighted workload formula to his or her current situation.

Interjudge reliability was their key to success. At a districtwide speech-language pathology meeting, the professionals compared and contrasted their weightings. Questions were answered and clarifications were given. Then the ad hoc committee presented eight case studies to the SLPs in the district. These professionals studied each case as it was presented on overhead slides and rated the workload associated with that case using the weighted formula. When all of the SLPs rated all eight cases similarly, the committee recognized that interjudge reliability had been attained The MCPASD ran a district-wide pilot project during the 2004–2005 school year. New contract language addressing the use of a weighted workload formula was developed for the school district's master contract. Each academic year, all of the SLPs in the school district collaborate with the elementary, middle school, and high school coordinators to create a weighted workload. All full-time equivalent (FTE) allocations are determined based on the weighted workload formula. For example, a caseload maximum may reflect the number 40; however, there may actually be only 37 students on the caseload because of the workload attached to those 37 students may yield a heavier weighting. Notbohm reported, "The administrators are beginning to understand the workload weighted system and to appreciate the value of the variety of services the SLPs provide with, for, and on behalf of students. It's amazing how successful we can be when the speech-language pathologists, administration, and teachers' union all work together" (H. Notbohm, personal communication, May 9, 2005). The MCPASD Elementary and Secondary Severity Rating Scales are reproduced, with permission, as Appendix 2–1 at the end of this chapter.

Summary

Caseload size has challenged school-based services since the first Education for All Handicapped Children Act was passed in 1975. The roles and responsibilities of the SLP have expanded over time as legal mandates have been added. In the post-IDEA '04 era, SLPs need to think in terms of workload responsibilities, not just direct service for the caseload. Research clearly shows negative effects of large caseload on student outcomes. SLPs must use a student-centered approach. It is not possible to apply one simple solution to caseload size, because each SLP's workload is uniquely defined by the IEPs of the students on that caseload. It is possible, however, to apply the same workload analysis approach to any caseload. A workload analysis approach to establishing caseload standards in the schools may appear time-consuming to the professional who is already overloaded. Nevertheless, a majority of the professionals who have used a workload analysis approach have found it to be useful, and many unique solutions and success stories have been documented.

Questions for Application and Review

1. How do large caseloads affect service delivery options used by SLPs in school-based programs?
2. How do large caseloads affect professional activities that are mandated?
3. How do large caseloads affect students' learning outcomes?
4. How do large caseloads affect burnout and attrition?
5. How do large caseloads affect compliance with IDEA '04?
6. How is *caseload* defined?
7. How is *workload* defined?
8. What are the four major premises of workload?
9. What are the four quadrants of a balanced workload?
10. Explain why one solution cannot be applied to every workload problem.

References

American Speech-Language-Hearing Association. (1984). Guidelines for caseload size and speech-language services in the schools. *Asha*, 53–58.

American Speech-Language-Hearing Association. (1991). A model for collaborative service delivery for students with language-learning disorders in the public schools. *Asha*, *33*(Suppl. 5), 44–50.

American Speech-Language-Hearing Association. (1996). Scope of practice in speech-language pathology. *Asha*, *38*(Suppl. 16), 16–20.

American Speech-Language-Hearing Association. (1999). *Guidelines for the roles and responsibilities of the school-based speech-language pathologist.* Available from www.asha.org/policy

American Speech-Language-Hearing Association. (2000a). *2000 schools survey.* Rockville, MD: Author.

American Speech-Language-Hearing Association. (2000b). *National data report 1999–2000: National outcomes measurement system.* Rockville, MD: Author.

American Speech-Language-Hearing Association. (2000c). *IDEA and your caseload. A template for eligibility and dismissal criteria for students ages 3 to 21.* Rockville, MD: Author.

American Speech-Language-Hearing Association. (2000d). Current state caseload sizes for school speech-language pathologists. *Perspectives on School-Based Issues Division 16 Newsletter, 1*(1), 19–20.

American Speech-Language-Hearing Association. (2000e). *Developing educationally relevant IEPs: A technical assistant document for speech-language pathologists.* Rockville, MD: Author.

American Speech-Language-Hearing Association. (2001a). *Roles and responsibilities of speech-language pathologists with respect to reading and writing in children and adolescents* [Position statement]. Available from www.asha.org/policy

American Speech-Language-Hearing Association. (2001b). Pre-kindergarten NOMS. *The Asha Leader, 6*(16), 25.

American Speech-Language-Hearing Association. (2002). *A workload analysis approach to caseload standards in schools.* Available from www.asha.org/policy.

American Speech-Language-Hearing Association. (2003). *Implementation guide: A workload analysis approach to caseload standards in schools.* Rockville, MD: Author.

American Speech-Language-Hearing Association. (2004). *Schools survey report: Caseload characteristics.* Rockville, MD: Author.

Banks, S., & Necco, E. (1990). The effects of special education category and type of training on job burnout in special education teachers. *Teacher Education and Special Education, 13*(3–4), 187–191.

Beck, A., & Dennis, M. (1997). Speech-language pathologists' and teachers' perceptions of classroom-based interventions. *Language, Speech, and Hearing Services in Schools, 28,* 146–153.

Blood, G. W., Swavely Ridenour, J., Thomas, E. A., & Qualls, C. D., (2002). Predicting job satisfaction among speech-language pathologists working in public schools. *Language, Speech, and Hearing Services in Schools, 33*(4), 282–290.

Chiang, B., & Rylance, B. (2000). *Wisconsin speech-language pathologists' caseloads: Reality and repercussions.* Oshkosh, WI: University of Wisconsin.

Cirrin, F., & Penner, S. (1995). Classroom-based and consultative service delivery models for language intervention. In M. Fey, J. Windsor, & S. Warren (Eds.), *Language intervention: Preschool through the elementary years.* Baltimore: Brookes.

Eger, D. (1992, November). Why now? Changing school speech-language service delivery. *Asha Magazine,* 40–41.

Ehren, B. (2000). Maintaining a therapeutic focus and sharing responsibility for student success: Keys to in-classroom speech-language services. *Language, Speech, and Hearing Services in Schools, 31,* 219–229.

Elksnin, L., & Capilouto, G. (1994). Speech-language pathologists' perceptions of integrated service delivery in school settings. *Language, Speech, and Hearing Services in Schools, 25,* 258–267.

Gillon, G. T. (2000). The efficacy of phonological awareness intervention. *Language, Speech, and Hearing Services in Schools, 31,* 126–141.

Goldberg, B. (1993, November). Recipe for tragedy: Personnel shortages in the public schools. *Asha Magazine,* 36–40.

Hart, B., & Risley, T. (1980). In vitro language intervention: Unanticipated general effects. *Journal of Applied Behavior Analysis, 13,* 407–432.

Hylton, J. (1987). *The role of the physical therapist and the occupational therapist in the school setting: Therapy in educational settings.* Portland, OR: Oregon Health Sciences University.

Johnson, B., & Meline, T. (1997). A survey of supervisor workload practices: Communication disorders programs in colleges. *Clinical Supervisor, 16*(1), 79–96.

Karr, S., & Schooling, T. (2001). *The impact of high caseloads on speech-language pathology services for children in schools.* Written Statement of the American Speech-Language-Hearing Association to the Virginia Board of Education. Rockville, MD: ASHA.

Keith, P. (1992, March). *School psychologists' use of time: Interventions and effectiveness.* Paper presented at the annual meeting of the National Association of School Psychologists, Philadelphia, PA. (ERIC Document Reproduction Service No. ED 348 605).

Lowenthal, B. (1981). Effect of small-group instruction on language-delayed preschoolers. *Exceptional Children, 48*(2), 178–179.

McCabe, J., Jenkins, J., Mills, P., Dale, P., Cole, K., & Pepler, L. (1996). Effects of play group variables on language use by preschool children with disabilities. *Journal of Early Intervention, 20*(4), 329–340.

Middleton/Cross Plains Area School District. (2005). *Speech-language severity rating scale: Elementary level*. Unpublished manuscript, Middleton, WI.

Middleton/Cross Plains Area School District. (2005). *Speech-language severity rating scale: Secondary level*. Unpublished manuscript, Middleton, WI.

Miller, M., & Potter, R. (1982, March). Professional burnout among speech-language pathologists. *Asha Magazine*, 177–180.

Mills, C., & Ivery, C. (1991). A strategy for workload management in child protective practice. *Child Welfare, 70*(1), 35–43.

National Joint Committee on Learning Disabilities. (1993, November). Reaction to "full inclusion": A reaffirmation of the right of students with learning disabilities to a continuum of services. *Asha Magazine*, 63.

Ohio Legislative Office of Education Oversight. (1999). *Availability of therapists to work in Ohio schools*. Columbus, OH: Author.

Olmstead, J. (1995). Itinerant personnel: A survey of caseloads and working conditions. *Journal of Visual Impairments & Blindness, 89*, 546–548.

Peters-Johnson, C. (1992, November). Professional practices perspective on caseloads in schools. *Asha Magazine*, 12.

Peters-Johnson, C. (1996). Action: School services. *Language, Speech, and Hearing Services in Schools, 27*, 185–186.

Peters-Johnson, C. (1998). Action: School services. *Language, Speech, and Hearing Services in Schools, 29*, 120–126.

Pezzei, C., & Oratio, A. (1991). A multivariate analysis of the job satisfaction of public school speech-language pathologists. *Language, Speech, and Hearing Services in Schools, 22*, 139–146.

Prelock, P. (2000). An intervention focus for inclusionary practice. *Language, Speech, and Hearing Services in Schools, 31*, 296–298.

Russ, S., Chiang, B., Rylance, B., & Bongers, J. (2001). Caseload in special education: An integration of research findings. *Exceptional Children, 67*(2), 161–172.

Rylance, B., Chiang, B., Russ, S., & Dobbs-Whitcomb, S. (1999). *Special education caseload and class size policies in the fifty states*. Madison, WI: Wisconsin State Department of Public Instruction.

Stein, T., Callaghan, J., McGee, L., & Douglas, S. (1990). A caseload-weighting formula for child welfare services. *Child Welfare, 69*(1), 33–42.

U.S. Congress (1975). *The Education for All Handicapped Children Act. Public Law 94-142*. Washington, DC: U.S. Government Printing Office.

U.S. Congress. (1997). *Individuals with Disabilities Education Act Amendments of 1997*. Washington, DC: U.S. Government Printing Office.

U.S. Department of Education. (2000). *Twenty second annual report to Congress on the implementation of the Individuals with Disabilities Education Act (IDEA)*. Washington, DC: U.S. Government Printing Office.

Warren, S., & Rogers-Warren, A. (1982). Language acquisition patterns in normal and handicapped children. *Topics in Early Childhood Special Education, 2*(2), 70–77.

Whitmire, K. (2000). Action: School services. *Language, Speech, and Hearing Services in Schools, 31*, 308–314.

Whitmire, K., Karr, S., & Mullen, R. (2000). Action: School services. *Language, Speech, and Hearing Services in Schools, 31*, 402–406.

Wisniewski, L., & Gargiulo, R. (1997). Occupational stress and burnout among special educators: A review of the literature. *Journal of Special Education, 31*(3), 325–346.

APPENDIX 2–1

Middleton/Cross Plains Area School District Speech-Language Severity Rating Scales

Speech-Language Severity Rating Scale: Elementary Level

Student's Name _____ D.O.B. _____

ID# _____ School _____ Grade _____

Program(s) _____ Form Completed by _____

This worksheet is for SLP use and is not intended to become part of the student's records.

Section 1: Results of Standardized, Criteria Reference, or Informal Testing
(for information purposes only)

Test	Date	Scores

Section 2: Factors That Influence the Need for Service
Score all that apply.

Begin student with a baseline factor of 1.0			**1.0**
No direct service	−0.3	Notes:	
Mild articulation needs only	−0.2	Notes:	
S/L services provided for 1 semester or less—not on a daily or weekly basis	−0.2	Notes:	
S/L program only (case management responsibilities)	+0.1	Notes:	
Individual intervention 3 or more times per week or phonology classroom	+0.1	Notes:	
Behavioral factors (demonstrates chronic and severe aggression, develop and/or implement behavior modification plans)	+0.1 +0.2	Notes:	
Academic support needs (such as curriculum/test modifications, planning with academic staff, tests read, etc.)	+0.1 +0.2	Notes:	
Consultation with outside agencies	+0.1	Notes:	
Adaptive/augmentative communication needs	+0.1	Notes:	
Specialized remediation program/materials needed (social language training, hearing impairment needs, picture schedules, etc.)	+0.2	Notes:	
Total:			

Speech-Language Severity Rating Scale: Secondary Level

Student's Name _____ D.O.B. _____

ID# _____ School _____ Grade _____

Program(s) _____ Form Completed by _____

This worksheet is for SLP use and is not intended to become part of the student's records.

Section 1: Results of Standardized, Criteria Reference, or Informal Testing
(for information purposes only)

Test	Date	Scores

Section 2: Factors That Influence the Need for Service
Score all that apply.

Begin student with a baseline factor of 1.0			1.0
No direct service	−0.4	Notes:	
Enrollment in 3 or more SEN/SWD academic classes that reduce academic support needs	−0.2	Notes:	
S/L services provided for 1 semester or less; not on a daily or weekly basis	−0.2	Notes:	
S/L program only (case management responsibilities)	+0.2	Notes:	
Behavioral factors (demonstrates chronic and severe aggression, develop and/or implement behavior modification plans)	+0.1 +0.2	Notes:	
Academic support needs (curriculum/test modifications, planning with academic staff, tests read, etc.)	+0.1 +0.2	Notes:	
Post-secondary transition needs (testing, applications, etc.)	+0.2	Notes:	
Adaptive-augmentative communication needs	+0.1	Notes:	
Specialized remediation program/materials needed (articulation, fluency, social language training, etc.)	+0.2	Notes:	
Total:			

S/L = speech-language.

SEN/SWD = special education needs

From Middleton-Cross Plains, WI Area School District. Reprinted with Permission.

Chapter 3

ASSESSMENT, EVALUATION, AND INDIVIDUALIZED EDUCATION PROGRAMS IN SCHOOLS

RELATED VOCABULARY

baseline data   Assessment data collected on a target behavior before the initiation of an intervention program.

buddy system   Pairing a student without a disability with a student who has a disability and allowing that child to offer assistance to the child with the disability during classroom learning activities.

emphatic stress   Use of voice intonation and patterns to focus on the critical aspects of a communicated message.

foster grandparent program   A volunteer program instituted by school districts in which senior citizens in the community receive a free school lunch in exchange for offering assistance to the teacher and children in a public school classroom.

local education agency (LEA)   A school or school district in which the child is enrolled for services.

mediation   A process by which an impartial third party facilitates discussion between two opposing parties for the sake of resolving the conflict.

multimodality   Using more than one of the five senses in the learning process.

The information presented in this chapter is based on mandates in the Individuals with Disabilities Education Improvement Act of 2004 (IDEA '04), Part B.

> **present level of educational and functional performance (PLEP)**
> A narrative summary of a child's strengths, interests, learning style, and challenges based on a synthesis of information acquired by an individualized education program team via the assessment and evaluation process.
>
> **youth-tutoring-youth program** A volunteer program instituted by school districts in which high school students who aspire to become educators use their study hall time to work with younger students under the supervision of the classroom teacher.

Introduction

Modern-day dispositions related to people with disabilities are reflected in the language of America's federal laws. IDEA '04 proclaimed:

Congress finds the following:

(1) Disability is a natural part of the human experience and in no way diminishes the right of individuals to participate in or contribute to society. Improving educational results for children with disabilities is an essential element of our national policy of ensuring equality of opportunity, full participation, independent living, and economic self-sufficiency for individuals with disabilities.

(2) Before the date of enactment of the Education for All Handicapped Children Act of 1975 (Public Law 94-142), the educational needs of millions of children with disabilities were not being fully met because

   (A) the children did not receive appropriate educational services;

   (B) the children were excluded entirely from the public school system and from being educated with their peers;

   (C) undiagnosed disabilities prevented the children from having a successful educational experience; or

   (D) a lack of adequate resources within the public school system forced families to find services outside the public school system.

(3) Since the enactment and implementation of the Education for All Handicapped Children Act of 1975, this title has been successful in ensuring children with disabilities and the families of such children access to a free appropriate public education and in improving educational results for children with disabilities.

(4) However, the implementation of this title has been impeded by low expectations, and an insufficient focus on applying replicable research on proven methods of teaching and learning for children with disabilities.

(5) Almost 30 years of research and experience has demonstrated that the education of children with disabilities can be made more effective by—

   (A) having high expectations for such children and ensuring their access to the general education curriculum in the regular classroom, to the maximum extent possible, in order to—

      (i) meet developmental goals and, to the maximum extent possible, the challenging expectations that have been established for all children; and

      (ii) be prepared to lead productive and independent adult lives, to the maximum extent possible;

   (B) strengthening the role and responsibility of parents and ensuring that families of such children have meaningful opportunities to participate in the education of their children at school and at home;

(C) coordinating this title with other local, educational service agency, State, and Federal school improvement efforts, including improvement efforts under the Elementary and Secondary Education Act of 1965, in order to ensure that such children benefit from such efforts and that special education can become a service for such children rather than a place where such children are sent;

(D) providing appropriate special education and related services, and aids and supports in the regular classroom, to such children, whenever appropriate;

(E) supporting high-quality, intensive preservice preparation and professional development for all personnel who work with children with disabilities in order to ensure that such personnel have the skills and knowledge necessary to improve the academic achievement and functional performance of children with disabilities, including the use of scientifically based instructional practices, to the maximum extent possible;

(F) providing incentives for whole-school approaches, scientifically based early reading programs, positive behavioral interventions and supports, and early intervening services to reduce the need to label children as disabled in order to address the learning and behavioral needs of such children;

(G) focusing resources on teaching and learning while reducing paperwork and requirements that do not assist in improving educational results." (Section 682 (c), IDEA '04)

The work of the U.S. Department of Education (2006), Wrightslaw (2004), the American Federation of Teachers, AFL-CIO (2005), the *Christian Science Monitor* (2005), and the National Education Association (2005) summarized the major components of IDEA '04. The mandates that public schools must provide a free appropriate public education (FAPE) in the least restrictive environment and follow detailed due process provisions

in order to obtain federal funding was preserved and strengthened by IDEA '04. Boehner and Castle (2005) provided a description of purpose for each part of the law. Part A of IDEA '04 contains the general provisions, including the purposes of the Act and definitions. Part B contains provisions relating to education of school-aged and preschool children, the funding formula, evaluation for services, eligibility determinations, individualized education programs (IEPs), and educational placements. It also contains detailed requirements for procedural safeguards (including the discipline provisions) as well as withholding of funds and judicial review. Part B also includes the Section 619 program, which provides services to children 3 to 5 years of age. Part C of IDEA specifies the requirement for early intervention and other services for infants and toddlers with disabilities and their families (from birth through age 3 years). Part D provides support for various national activities designed to improve the education of children with disabilities, including personnel preparation activities, technical assistance, and special education research. The assessment, evaluation, and IEP development mandated by IDEA '04 are described in this chapter.

Prereferral

The assessment and evaluation process begins in the general education arena. Before a student may be referred for special education or related services, the public school must document that all regular education options have been attempted and that the student is still not successful in the general education curriculum. Many public schools have prereferral building-team meetings that are held on a weekly, biweekly, or monthly basis. Regular education teachers and special education personnel meet and brainstorm regarding various options relevant to the needs of each student who is not being successful in the general education curriculum. Each regular education option is pursued; the results are observed; and documentation is compiled and reviewed before a referral for special education and related services is considered. Under Part B (E), Rules of Construction, screening conducted by a teacher or specialist is not considered part of an evaluation for eligibility for special education and related services. Thus, screening may be conducted without parent permission. Presented next are a few examples of regular education options that may be implemented before a referral for special education or related services may be made:

- **Youth-tutoring-youth program:** High school students who are interested in pursuing a career in education volunteer to work with younger students who are not experiencing success in their academics. The high school students volunteer during a study hall, before school, or after school.
- **Foster grandparent program:** Senior citizens volunteer to work with students who are not experiencing success in their academics. In some cases the senior citizens receive a free hot lunch each day that they volunteer.
- **Buddy system:** The student who is not experiencing success in the classroom is paired with another student who serves as a peer tutor.
- **Changes in the classroom environment:** Modifications are made to the acoustical characteristics of the classroom to decrease the amount of noise distractions. Such modifications may include covering the floor with carpet, adding sound absorbing material to the walls, installing acoustical ceiling tile, adding materials that absorb sound to the walls, placing draperies on the windows, and sealing classroom doors with felt or vinyl sound stripping, and using a frequency modulated (FM) system. Work centers with study carrels or dividers brought into the classroom and making ear plugs available to the students may be other acoustic modifications considered.
- **Changes in the teaching style:** The general education teacher(s) apply evidence-based, research-based strategies that have not been used before. Examples of strategies to try are increasing redundancy of instruction; using **multimodality** forms of instruction or student response forms, or both; adding visuals and graphic organizers; reviewing relevant past material as a part of the transition to new concepts; providing pretutoring; coordinating home activities for reinforcement of major concepts; using a slower rate of speech; using increased **emphatic stress** on target concepts; simplifying directions; simplifying vocabulary; frequently checking the student's comprehension; employing a proactive, consistent behavior management program; and using computer software to provide massed practice.

Such strategies must be implemented in the general education setting and the results documented before a referral. IDEA '04 strengthened the prereferral process and encouraged schools that have a disproportionate number of students of color enrolled in special education and related services to expand their prereferral systems. IDEA '04 proclaimed:

(10) (A) The Federal Government must be responsive to the growing needs of an increasingly diverse society. (B) America's ethnic profile is rapidly changing. In 2000, 1 of every 3 persons in the United States was a member of a minority group or was limited English proficient. (C) Minority children comprise an increasing percentage of public school students. (D) With such changing demographics, recruitment efforts for special education personnel should focus on increasing the participation of minorities in the teaching profession in order to provide appropriate role models with sufficient knowledge to address the special education needs of these students. (11) (A) The limited English proficient population is the fastest growing in our Nation, and the growth is occurring in many parts of our Nation. (B) Studies have documented apparent discrepancies in the levels of referral and placement of limited English proficient children in special edu-

cation. (C) Such discrepancies pose a special challenge for special education in the referral of, assessment of, and provision of services for, our Nation's students from non-English language backgrounds. (12) (A) Greater efforts are needed to prevent the intensification of problems connected with mislabeling and high dropout rates among minority children with disabilities. (B) More minority children continue to be served in special education than would be expected from the percentage of minority students in the general school population. (C) African-American children are identified as having mental retardation and emotional disturbance at rates greater than their White counterparts. (D) In the 1998–1999 school year, African-American children represented just 14.8 percent of the population aged 6 through 21, but comprised 20.2 percent of all children with disabilities. (E) Studies have found that schools with predominately White students and teachers have placed disproportionately high numbers of their minority students into special education. (13) (A) As the number of minority students in special education increases, the number of minority teachers and related services personnel produced in colleges and universities continues to decrease. (B) The opportunity for full participation by minority individuals, minority organizations, and historically Black Colleges and Universities in awards for grants and contracts, boards of organizations receiving assistance under this title, peer review panels, and training of professionals in the area of special education is essential to obtain greater success in the education of minority children with disabilities. (14) As the graduation rates for children with disabilities continue to climb, providing effective transition services to promote successful post-school employment or education is an important measure of accountability for children with disabilities." [Section 682 (c)]

Referral for Evaluation for Special Education and Related Services

Physicians, nurses, psychologists, social workers, administrators of social agencies, and school personnel are required to make a referral for evalua-

tion for special education and related services when they suspect that a student has a disability. Any professional whose position allows observation of or interaction with the student, however, may make a referral. Before the referral is submitted, the student's parent or legal guardian must be informed that the referral is being made. When the **local education agency** (LEA) receives the referral, the 60-day timeline from receipt of referral to sending placement notice begins. School districts must have written procedures describing the referral process. Parents and legal guardians must be informed of their legal rights at the time the referral is made. IDEA '04 stated that informed parental consent must be obtained before an evaluation is conducted and also before providing special education and related services to the child. If the parent fails to provide consent, however, the LEA may pursue the initial evaluation by following procedures described in Section 615. If the parent refuses to provide consent for the child to receive special education and related services, the LEA is not required to convene an IEP meeting. If the child is a ward of the state, the LEA must make a reasonable attempt to inform the parents about an initial evaluation, IEP development, and placement unless the parents' whereabouts are unknown or the parents' rights have been terminated or subrogated by a judge in accordance with state law.

The Individualized Education Program Team

When a referral is made, the LEA appoints an IEP team. This team includes the following:

- The parent or legal guardian of the student. The parent or legal guardian is considered an equal team member and participants on the IEP team.
- At least one general education teacher who is currently involved in the student's education.
- At least one special education teacher trained in the area related to the student's known or suspected disability.

■ An LEA representative who is qualified to provide or supervise the provision of special education and related services; is knowledgeable about the general curriculum; is knowledgeable about the availability of LEA resources; and is authorized to commit LEA resources. This individual may fill another role on the IEP team if he or she meets the requirements for another role.

■ A person who can interpret the instructional implications of evaluation results. This person also may fill another role.

■ Other individuals at the discretion of the parents, legal guardians, or LEA, including related services personnel.

■ The student, whenever appropriate. The student must be invited to any IEP meeting at which transition services are discussed. Transition services must be considered for any student 16 to 21 years of age.

Assessment Activities

After an initial referral has been made, the LEA provides the parent or legal guardian with a notice of the referral. The notice includes the names of those whom the LEA has appointed as IEP team participants and the qualifications of the participants. The IEP team, including the parents or legal guardians, reviews the existing data and decides whether additional data must be collected in order to determine whether the student has a disability. The IEP team must review existing data, including information provided by the parent or legal guardian, previous interventions and their effects, current classroom-based assessments, and observations by teachers and others. Existing data also may include any information from outside sources such as assessment data for a student in transition from a "birth-to-3" program or Head Start program. An IEP meeting to review the existing data is not required; however, the IEP team may decide to hold such a meeting. If the IEP team finds that no additional data are needed, the LEA notifies the parents or legal guardians in writing of the find-

ing and the reasons for it. The next step is to notify the parents of an IEP team meeting, when a determination will be made about whether the child has an impairment that results in a disability, and whether this disability warrants special education or related services based on existing data. IDEA '04 allows the parent or legal guardian to participate in such a meeting via video- or teleconferencing. With any disagreement between the parent and the LEA about whether additional data are needed that cannot be resolved, the parent or legal guardian, or LEA may pursue **mediation**, due process, or complaints. Mediation is an option at every stage of the IEP process. As proclaimed in IDEA '04 Section 682 (c), parents and schools should try to resolve any disagreement in a positive and constructive way. Assessment of the student must be nondiscriminatory and standardized tests may be used only in the ways they were designed and apply only to the populations they were designed to assess. Parents' permission is required before new tests or other assessment tools are used. The child must be assessed in all the areas of suspected disability.

Evaluation Process

Decision making about an individual student is based on the judgment of the IEP team members, including the parent, who must work collaboratively. All evaluations must include the following:

■ Multiple data sources such as teachers, parents, students, and other service providers familiar to the student

■ Multiple types of data that are quantitative and qualitative in nature

■ Multiple types of tools and procedures such as standardized measures, authentic assessment, dynamic assessment, and alternative methods of assessment

■ Multiple environments such as classrooms, playground, community settings, and home

Response to learning is a possible consideration in evaluation of a child suspected of having a learning disability. All IEP team members who conduct new tests or other assessments procedures must submit a summary of their findings, which is made available to all team participants at the IEP team meeting. The summary of findings is in writing; is about one page in length; and must be understandable to all IEP team participants. Each summary of findings becomes part of the evaluation report and is not a "stand-alone" document. It is not legal for an IEP team member to make recommendations about whether a student meets eligibility criteria based solely on his or her individual summary of findings. Evaluating the assessment data must be a collaborative team effort.

Evaluation Report

The IEP team documents the evaluation findings in an evaluation report. This report must include the following elements:

- A review of the existing data
- Findings from any additional assessment tools administered
- Determination of eligibility
- Whether the student has an impairment based on eligibility criteria
- Whether the impairment results in a disability
- Whether the disability warrants special education or related services
- Whether accommodations are needed under Section 504 of the Rehabilitation Act
- Additional required documentation if the child was evaluated for a learning disability: For a student suspected of having a specific learning disability, each IEP team member must certify in writing whether the report reflects his or her conclusion; if it does not, the IEP team member must submit a separate statement presenting his or her conclusions.
- Additional required documentation if the student was evaluated for a visual impairment or if a student with a visual impairment requires Braille

- Consideration of the student's communication needs
- Consideration of the student's needs for assistive technology or related services

The IEP team collaboratively creates a **present level of educational and functional performance** (PLEP) statement that reflects the student's strengths, interests, learning style, and challenges (or needs). **Baseline data** related to the student's needs must be reported; in addition, a statement about how the student's needs adversely affect his or her ability to make progress in the general education curriculum must be included. Each need must be translated into a goal on the IEP. The baseline data related to the need also must be incorporated into the goal on the IEP as the baseline for that goal.

Reevaluation: General Provisions

Reevaluations are conducted at the request of the student's parent or teacher, when conditions warrant, and at least once every 3 years. IDEA '04 allowed implementation of a 3-year IEP for a student between the ages of 18 to 21. The procedures for reevaluation are essentially the same as for initial evaluations. Prior to beginning a reevaluation, the LEA provides the parent with written notice. This notice informs the parent that the LEA intends to reevaluate the student and the reason for the reevaluation. The notice also includes the IEP team participants, in addition to the parent and child (if appropriate), who have been appointed by the LEA, their names, and qualifications. The IEP team reviews existing data, including the following:

- Existing assessment data
- Information provided by the parents
- Previous interventions and their effects
- Current classroom-based information
- Observations and interviews

On reevaluation, if after reviewing existing data, the IEP team determines that no additional data are needed, the LEA notifies the parent in writing of the findings and the reasons for it, and the parent's right to request assessment to determine whether the student continues to demonstrate a disability. Providing the parents or legal guardians with written notice is a statutory requirement, even though they are IEP team participants and thus already know the decision.

If additional data are needed, the parent is notified, and a description of the types of tests and other assessment tools to be conducted and the names (if known) and qualifications of examiners are provided. Parental consent is needed before administration of new tests or assessments or application of other evaluation materials. Consent need not be obtained if the LEA has taken reasonable measures and parents fail to respond. Such cases differ from those in which the parent refuses to give consent. Consideration of progress made is taken into account at the 3-year reevaluation. On the basis of a review of existing data (and the results of new tests and other evaluation materials if administered), the IEP team makes the following determinations:

- Whether the student has or continues to have impairment
- Whether the impairment results in a disability
- Whether the disability warrants special education and related services
- The present levels of performance and educational needs of the student
- Whether the student needs special education
- Whether additions or modifications to the special education and related services are needed to enable the student to meet the measurable, annual goals specified on the student's IEP and, if needed, to participate as appropriate in the general education curriculum

The Individualized Education Program

The IEP team creates a PLEP based on the evaluation results. The PLEP must include the student's strengths, interests, learning style, and needs (or challenges). The needs must be written in observ-able, measurable terms and must show baseline performance. The PLEP must include a statement about how the student's needs are interfering with progress in the general education curriculum. Each need that is identified in the PLEP must be addressed as a goal on the IEP. Each goal must connect to the general education curriculum standards and include seven specific elements:

1. *Time frame*: The length of time it will take the student to achieve the goal. The time-frame must not exceed one academic year.
2. *Condition*: The modifications and accommodations that will be made to help the student become successful.
3. *Direction of behavior*: Whether the child will increase, decrease, or maintain a specific behavior. Maintenance of a behavior is rarely used but sometimes appropriate for a student with a degenerative disease or medically fragile condition.
4. *Target behavior*: What the student is expected to achieve.
5. *Baseline*: The student's demonstrated skills documented in the evaluation of assessment data. This is taken from the PLEP as related to the identified need.
6. *Criteria*: This category reflects how much progress the student is expected to achieve within the designated time frame.
7. *Setting*: This describes the least restrictive environment that is appropriate for the individual student.

The following example IEP goal, written in accordance with IDEA '04, includes these seven elements:

Goal: Within 36 weeks, when given auditory, visual, and tactile cues, the student will increase speech intelligibility from 40% to 70% while reading a textbook aloud in the classroom setting. (*Note*: 36 weeks = 180 school days or one academic year.)

IDEA '04 no longer requires benchmarks or objectives to be written on the IEP unless the student does not participate in statewide or district-wide assessment programs. Nevertheless, educators may continue to write short-term objectives or benchmarks as a way of reporting progress toward the IEP goal.

A Historical Perspective: Ongoing Evolution of Individualized Education Programs

It is useful for the SLP to know how IEPs have evolved over the years, because not all school districts have kept pace with the changes. Thus, the SLP may encounter IEPs that look very different when a child transfers from another state or even another school within the same district. In an effort to continue the quest for quality, as well as equality, of services for children in special education and related services, advocates and parents have kept a focus on goal writing since IDEA was authorized in 1990. Before 1990, IEP goals were written in general terms and used nonspecific language such as *improve*, *enhance*, or *develop*. Objectives were used instead of benchmarks. At least two objectives were written for each goal. Each objective contained a condition, target behavior, and criteria. No baseline was included, no direction of behavior was required, and the accountability for the criteria was nonspecific (e.g., based on teacher-made test, classroom observation, or parent report). The following example presents a goal and two benchmarks written in the 1990s style:

Goal: The student will improve oral communication skills.

Objective: When given a model-imitation task, the student will produce a mean length of utterance of 3.5, 60% of the time based on classroom observations.

Objective: When given an elicitation task, the student will produce a mean length of utterance of 3.5, 75% of the time as measured by a teacher-made test.

When IDEA was reauthorized in 1997, more emphasis was placed on the LRE. IEP goals had to be curriculum based and reflect the LRE. Bench-marks were allowed instead of objectives because the goal had to relate to education standards delineated by each state. The IEP goals had to include a direction of behavior (e.g., increase, decrease, maintain). The goals had to include baseline data taken from the PLEP. The goals also had to include criteria that were observable and measurable. The benchmarks had to be written in observable, measurable terms. The following example presents a goal and two benchmarks written in the IDEA '97 style:

Goal: When given visual cues, Juan will increase speech intelligibility from 40% to 70% while engaged in classroom communication learning activities.

Benchmark: Juan will produce /k, g/ sounds at the beginning and end of words in 8 out of 10 trials while reading a 200 word passage from a grade level text that has highlighted letters.

Benchmark: Juan will produce /k, g/ sounds in the initial, medial, and final positions of words and in consonant blends in 8 out of 10 trials while reading a 200-word passage from a grade level text that does not have highlighted letters.

IDEA '04 specifies that not every IEP team member must be present at every IEP meeting if the parents and LEA agree that the member's attendance is not necessary. Also, an IEP may be modified without convening a meeting if the parents and IEP team members agree to the changes. Court cases continue to shape the extent and quality of special education and related services and provisions within the IEP. An excellent resource for keeping abreast of new changes is the IDEA website (http://idea.gov).

Summary

Although the SLP working in a medical setting or private sector may diagnose and treat an impairment, the process is not so simple in the school setting. The assessment and evaluation process is complex and based on mandates in federal law and state regulations. It is not legal for one professional to make determinations, nor is it legal for one assessment tool to be used in the evaluation process. Parental rights and due process must be honored. The process must be nondiscriminatory. The process begins with prereferral activities. The IEP team must include the parent or legal guardian as an equal partner. The IEP team must determine whether a child has an impairment based on eligibility criteria, whether that impairment results in a disability, and whether that disability warrants special education or related services. The evaluation report must reflect the student's present level of performance. The PLEP must include the student's strengths, interests, and learning style as well as needs. The educational needs must be written in observable, measurable terms and must show how the disability interferes with the student's ability to make progress in the general education curriculum. Each need identified in the PLEP must be translated into a goal on the IEP. The baseline data for each goal must be taken from the PLEP. The IEP goals must be curriculum based and must reflect educational standards established by the state.

Questions for Application and Review

1. What is the first step in the assessment and evaluation process?
2. What is the responsibility of the SLP if the parents or legal guardians refuse to give permission to evaluate?
3. What is the definition of *assessment*?
4. What is the definition of *evaluation*?
5. What must be included in the PLEP statement?
6. How do the baseline data reported in the PLEP relate to the IEP goal?
7. How has the writing of IEP goals changed over time?
8. When does an IEP goal written after IDEA '04 have to include benchmarks or objectives?
9. What are the important parts of a goal?
10. Why is it important to avoid professional jargon in writing goals?

References

American Federation of Teachers, AFL-CIO. (2005). *Individuals with Disabilities Education Improvement Act 2004 summary*. Retrieved January 20, 2005, from http://www.aft.org

Boehner, J., & Castle, M. (2005). *Individuals with Disabilities Education Act (IDEA) guide to frequently asked questions*. Committee on Education and the Workforce. Retrieved January 20, 2005, from http://edworkforce.house.gov/issues/109th/education/idea/ideafaq.pdf

Christian Science Monitor. (2004). *A special compromise on education*. Retrieved January 20, 2005, from http://csmonitor.com/2004/1122/p11s01-legn.html

National Education Association. *Congress reauthorizes IDEA: NEA wins key changes*. Retrieved January 20, 2005, from http://www.nea.org/specialed/reautho rization.html

U. S. Congress Public Law 108-446, 118 Stat 2647, The Individuals with Disabilities Education Improvement Act of 2004, Part B Sec 611–615.

U.S. Department of Education. (2006). *Building the legacy: IDEA 2004*. Part B Sec 611–615 Retrieved September 4, 2007, from http://idea.ed.gov

Wrightslaw. (2004). *How will IEPs change under IDEA 2004?* Retrieved January 20, 2005, from http://www.wrightslaw.com

Chapter 4

SPEECH-LANGUAGE SERVICE DELIVERY FORMATS USED IN PUBLIC SCHOOLS: INTERVENTION APPROACHES

RELATED VOCABULARY

cognitive-developmental   Referring to an intervention approach in which the speech-language pathologist assesses the child's stage of development, based on piagetian theory, and then structures the learning environment and activities to enhance the child's growth of perception, memory, imagination, conception, judgment, and reason within that stage.

consultation model   A service delivery model in which the speech-language pathologist provides ideas for accommodations or modifications that may be implemented by others to meet the individualized needs of a student.

decontextualized   Describing interventions or situations in which all context clues are removed.

direct instruction   A teaching style that involves scripted interactions between the teacher and students with drill and practice activities.

dyad   An interaction unit consisting of two people.

heterogeneous   Grouping students who have different developmental levels, needs, deficits, or learning styles.

Hodson cycles approach   An intervention approach and service delivery model, developed by Barbara Hodson, that is designed to facilitate intelligible speech patterns in children with expressive phonological impairment (EPI).

homogeneous   Grouping students who have similar developmental levels, needs, deficits, or learning styles.

interpersonal communication   Communication between two or more people.

metalinguistic   Referring to the conscious awareness of using language, recognizing multiple meanings, drawing inferences, understanding figurative language, planning discourse, and organizing components of language.

milieu language teaching   An intervention approach that requires the speech-language pathologist to (1) select language targets at the appropriate developmental level, (2) structure the environment to increase the likelihood of student-initiated communication, (3) encourage expansion of child-initiated utterances, and (4) reinforce the child's communication attempts with access to desired objects or attention.

multisensory   Describing intervention strategies that activate more than one of the five senses in the learning process.

phonics   A method of teaching reading that focuses on the study of sounds associated with alphabet letters or the groupings of alphabet letters (graphemes) or into syllables.

phonology   The selected sound patterns used in any given language to construct its words and sentences based on a linguistic rule system; also, the study of sound in language.

phonological awareness   The ability to identify, blend, separate, and manipulate the sound patterns within a language.

psychogenic   Resulting from emotional conflict.

responsiveness-to-intervention   An approach to assessment by which the speech-language pathologist or other educator uses effective, efficient research-based instruction techniques and then analyzes how the student responds to those techniques. A problem-solving framework is used to identify and address the student's unique learning style or learning deficits.

scaffolding   An intervention approach in which the speech-language pathologist asks guided questions to bring the student to a higher level of understanding than that attainable without such assistance.

script training   An intervention approach in which the speech-language pathologist helps the student practice routine phrases or dialogues that commonly are used during activities of daily living or in specific contexts.

self-contained Describing a service delivery model in which students with disabilities receives special education and or support services in an environment that does not allow the students to interact with nondisabled peers.

semantic map A visual diagram, outline, or graphic organizer that enables the student to generate relevant information about contexts, attributes, comparisons, contrasts, part-whole relationships, inductive reasoning, deductive reasoning, sequence, cause and effect, prediction, analogies, hierarchy, or classification.

shared storybook reading An intervention approach in which the speech-language pathologist reads a story aloud while engaging the child or children listening in a discussion that is rich in language-enhancing techniques.

situated pragmatics An intervention approach in which the speech-language pathologist focuses on teaching the language needed in specific social routines.

Introduction

When speech-language pathology services were first introduced into public schools in the early 1900s, the itinerant "pull-out" approach was the only service delivery format used. Students were pulled out of their classrooms individually or in small groups to receive services designed to cure their speech impediments, voice problems, and stammering (as it was then called). This *pull-out model* is still used today (ASHA, 2001a, 2001b; Chiang & Rylance, 2000; Peters-Johnson, 1996, 1998). The pull-out service delivery program format is most likely to be used when the caseload size is large. Caseload size heavily influences the type of service delivery approach (ASHA, 2000, 2002a, 2002b, 2002c; Karr & Schooling, 2001; Whitmire, Karr, & Mullen, 2000). Of note, however, when a workload analysis approach to caseload standards in schools is used (ASHA, 2003; Annett, 2002, 2003, 2004; Cirrin et al., 2003; Moore, 2004; Whitmire, 2003) and the mandate for providing services in the least restrictive environment is honored (Chaney & Burk, 1998; Haynes, 1990; Kuder, 1997;

Lowe, 1993; McCormick, Frome Loeb, & Schiefelbusch, 1997; McCoy, 1995; Merritt & Culatta, 1998; Neidecker & Blosser, 1993; O'Connell, 1997; Oyer, Hall, & Haas, 1994; Paul, 1995; Simon, 1991; Taylor, 1992; Villa & Thousand, 1995; Whitmire & Dublinske, 2003), new and different service delivery approaches emerge.

The modern-day SLP must consider the individual needs of each student when selecting the appropriate service delivery approach. No single approach is adequate to meet the needs of all students. In general, service delivery approaches used with early childhood and elementary-aged students tend to be **cognitive-developmental** in nature. Direct skills are taught. For example, when working with an elementary aged student who does not have classification skills, the SLP directly teaches curriculum-based, standards-based classification skills. Intervention focuses on learning how things are the same and how things are different; classifying objects by perception (e.g., size, shape, color, texture); classifying objects by location (e.g., things found in the kitchen, bathroom, or garage); classifying objects by function (e.g., things that cut, things that fly, things that may be used for writing) and classifying objects by category (e.g., animal, mineral, plant).

When providing services to middle school students, rather than using a **direct instruction** approach, the SLP may shift to a strategy-based approach. For example, the middle school student may be taught compensatory classification strategies such as color-coding a science book cover with the same-colored notebook and the same-colored folder. Classification strategies can be intertwined with teaching strategies for note taking, test taking, time management, stress management, metacognitive self-reflection, and self-advocacy. The SLP and the student may use homework assignments from the general education curriculum and intertwine the achievement of individualized education program (IEP) goals into completion of the classroom assignments. When employed effectively, this approach is very different from tutoring. Specific goals are targeted; specific clinical strategies are employed; and progress toward those goals is documented in observable, measurable terms. The goal is not simply to finish the homework or provide tutorial services.

At the high school level, the SLP may focus on teaching functional life skills, social skills, and more strategies for compensating. For example, when working with a high school-aged student who continues to struggle with classification skills, the SLP may shadow the student in community-based settings and teach functional, life skills that are relevant to the job site or home. For example, the student may be taught how to recognize hazardous materials versus materials that are not hazardous, or to identify the difference between materials that are dangerous from those that are not. The student can learn what is safe and what is not safe in the job and home environments.

Selecting Program Formats

The foregoing examples summarize general trends in intervention approaches. However, they are not to be construed as "hard-and-fast" rules. It is very possible for all three approaches to be used at all three academic levels. The decision regarding which intervention approach is most appropriate for each student rests with the IEP team. The approach must be tailored to meet the individual child's needs. A specific approach should never be adopted merely because it is administratively convenient or is the only approach readily available. For example, a high school student who requires individualized, direct intervention for a fluency disorder should not be forced into a functional life skills program just because that is the only program the high school SLP is easily able to provide or the one that the administration is most easily able to schedule.

Self-Contained Program Model

Haynes, Moran, and Pindzola (1990) described the **self-contained** classroom as one in which the SLP serves as the specialized teacher and is responsible for the total curriculum. Self-contained classrooms were very popular in the 1990s and used widely at the early childhood and elementary school levels, where an early childhood specialist and an SLP often team taught with support staff. The mandate for least restrictive environment, however, caused many self-contained classrooms to be phased out. In the post-IDEA '04 era, the self-contained classroom model may be used only if the IEP team can justify that it is the most appropriate setting to meet the needs of the student.

The **phonology** classroom is one example of the self-contained classroom model that still exists. Phonology classrooms typically are used with preschool children who exhibit severe phonological deficits and who have no other needs. Neidecker and Blosser (1993) described the phonology classroom as a block system in which the child is seen four or five times a week for a concentrated block of time, usually 4 to 6 weeks. McLearie and Gross (1996) documented that when the block system is used with articulation cases, it results in service to a greater number of children; a higher dismissal rate from special education programs; a reduction in the length of time children need to be enrolled; greater carryover of improvement;

closer relationships among the SLP, school personnel, and parents; higher student motivation over a longer period of time; and less time spent in review activities. Conversely, McLearie and Gross documented that the block system was not adequate when problems of a **psychogenic** nature were concurrent; when it resulted in scheduling conflicts with other academic activities; and when it created an inability to share classroom space with other programs.

The **Hodson cycles approach** is an intervention approach that can be implemented in a self-contained phonology classroom, as well as under other arrangements. As described by Bowen (1998), the theoretical base for the Hodson cycles approach is that phonological acquisition is a complex, developmental interaction among motoric, perceptual, conceptual, and cognitive-linguistic abilities at the **interpersonal communication** level. This complex interaction is needed for the child to develop age-appropriate phonological patterns.

An example of how a Hodson cycles self-contained classroom might operate follows:

A group of 15 four-year-olds who demonstrate multiple phonological process errors come to a school classroom 2 hours per day, 4 days per week for 6 weeks. The classroom is staffed by three SLPs. A specific phonological process is intensely targeted as the children engage in high-interest, developmentally appropriate activities.

The children begin their session with a 15-minute large-group activity in which the targeted phonological pattern (e.g., /st/ clusters) is introduced. Then the large group is divided into three smaller groups, with five students per group. Each small group completes three different activities in rotation. At one table, the small group receives auditory bombardment. The children listen through headphones as the SLP says words containing /st/ clusters into a frequency modulated (FM) system. The children color pictures of objects that contain /st/ clusters while listening. At another table, the children *st*aple *st*ickers onto *st*ars as the second SLP incorporates model-imitation or -elicited practice

of the target sound. At a third table, the students *st*ick *st*ickers on a *st*ar while the third SLP provides linguistic input with a focus on the target phonological target.

The three groups rotate activities every 15 to 20 minutes until all three groups of children have experienced all three activities. A 15-minute bathroom break is scheduled, during which the children walk down the hall by *st*epping on pictures of words that start with /st/ clusters that have been taped to the floor. The children return to the classroom and play an "I Spy" game finding /st/ cluster objects hidden around the room. The three groups come together for a snack of *st*ar cookies with *st*icky frosting, *st*ar-shaped sandwiches, and *st*rawberry milk that they must *st*ir with a wooden *st*ir-*st*ick. Then the children all move to the floor, and an SLP reads aloud a book loaded with /s/ clusters; meanwhile, the other two SLPs write notes home to the parents and compile activities for home study. The session ends with a 15-minute good-bye time, when the students *st*ick the *st*ory and other home carryover activities into their respective *st*ar bags.

The entire 2-hour time block, divided into eight 15-minute sessions, provides the SLPs with opportunities to enhance each child's motoric, perceptual, conceptual, and cognitive-linguistic capacities at the interpersonal level. A second group of 15 students go through the same routine during an afternoon session. The two groups of 15 students take a break from services (cycle off) after 6 weeks so that two other groups can cycle on.

The three SLPs share a caseload of 60 students who cycle on or off for 6 weeks of intensive work and then are engaged in carryover home programs in between their cycles. Each SLP is the case manager for 20 students. The students typically are enrolled in the program for one semester. Thus, each SLP may have a caseload of 40 across the academic year.

The reader is referred to the work of Hodson and Paden (1992) and Hodson (2007) for more in-depth information about the cycles approach.

Resource Room Model

Haynes, Moran, and Pindzola (1990) described a resource room as one in which the SLP provides individual intervention, group intervention, or a combination of both. The resource room approach is used more widely at the middle school level but also may be implemented at the elementary and high school levels. The students spend most of their time in general education classrooms and go to the resource room one or two periods per day. The SLP typically uses a strategy-based remediation approach and intertwines each student's IEP goal(s) into the completion of homework assignments from the general education curriculum. Audiotaped classroom materials, highlighted textbooks, specialized computer software programs, simplified directions, modified lighting, modified furniture, distraction-free study areas, and dictionaries with enlarged print are some examples of the adaptations and modifications that may be provided in a resource room. At the middle school and high school levels, the student may receive course credit for time spent in the resource room if curriculum-based goals are achieved. In such cases, a course grade may be entered on the report card.

The SLP uses specific clinical strategies such as **milieu language teaching**, **scaffolding**, **semantic maps**, social routines, **script training**, and situational pragmatics while interacting with the students. McCormick, Frome Lobe, and Schiefel-busch (1997) described the outcomes of milieu teaching as increased frequency of communicative behaviors; production of longer and more complex utterances; and expression of familiar functions with more advanced forms. These positive outcomes are achieved through scaffolding or supporting a student in such a way that he or she can understand and use language at a level that is more complex than could be grasped or produced independently. Semantic maps, or mind maps, often are used as visual cues to help the student outline, brainstorm, or generate ideas related to a topic. Routines with a social purpose are practiced multiple times. Scripts of familiar events or routines are used to help the student understand the order of events. The SLP also may provide **situated pragmatics**, instruction that provides contextual support in social settings.

The following example shows how a resource room operates:

> For one period each day, instead of a study hall, 40 seventh-grade students who have language-based learning disabilities go the SLP resource room in groups of 10. The SLP works with the group to teach strategies and develop such skills as learning to (1) read the end of chapter questions before reading the chapter contents from a classroom science book; (2) focus on the bold print in the textbook to identify the major concepts of the lesson; (3) use a glossary, table of contents, and highlighted text; (4) identify the topic sentence of a paragraph; (5) use a semantic map or mind map to organize major concepts; (6) speak and write with longer sentences and greater sentence complexity; (7) use note-taking strategies; (8) use test-taking strategies; (9) be aware of one's own learning style; (10) organize materials, space, and time; (11) access information by developing computer literacy and dictionary skills; and (12) think critically and ask and answer questions. The SLP works with 10 students per grade during four periods of the day, has one period per day to conduct other workload activities, and devotes two periods per day to inclusive practices and classroom observations across all four grade levels. The students receive a credit and grade on their report card for their progress toward their individualized, curriculum-based goals on their IEPs.

Consultation Model

As documented by Haynes, Moran, and Pindzola (1990), when using a **consultative-collaborative model**, the SLP develops the intervention plan and then trains another educator, or para- educator, in how to implement the plan. Many self-contained early childhood programs have been replaced with the consultation service model as a result of the strong focus on the mandate for the least restrictive environment set forth in IDEA '04. When using the consultation model, the SLP may go to community-based settings and work with parents and staff, who incorporate the IEP goals into the children's daily living activities. Parents usually are involved. Intervention services may be incorporated into center-based, home-based, or day care–based settings. Using a combination of settings often proves to be the most effective.

The Rochester Hearing and Speech Center (RHSC) in Rochester, New York, uses the consultative-collaborative model. Feeney, Riddle, and Benedict (2000) document that the consultation model requires a systematic process of planning, problem solving, and data collection; must be goal directed; must not be imposed by an expert, but must be embraced voluntarily by all interested parties; must include all team members as co-equals; requires reciprocity among team members; involves joint problem definition and shared decision making; and results in optimal outcomes only through shared responsibility. In a consultative-collaborative model, the SLP provides information about child language development; the critical role of teachers and caregivers in supporting language development; training that empowers the caregivers; and feedback related to the reports and observations of teachers and caregivers.

RHSC uses a five-step model in the consultative-collaborative process. First, during a general orientation, the SLP explains the process to and helps create the attitude that the problem can be resolved. (*Example*: Teacher: "Sondra won't talk in class; she hits the other children to get her way." In this case the SLP explains that Sondra may be hitting because she does not have the words to describe her desires. By enhancing Sondra's language skills, she may also develop a less aggressive interaction style with her peers.) The second step is problem definition and formulation. All parties work together to clearly define all aspects of the problem in operational terms. (*Example*: Teacher: "Sondra says two or three phrases and about 10 single words in an hour

when she is enjoying play time, but says nothing at lunch or circle time. She does not use words to make requests"). The third step is the generation of alternatives. During this step, the parties brainstorm all possible solutions to the problem. (*Example*: Teacher: "We could have our volunteer spend 15 minutes a day with Sondra during playtime.") The fourth step is a process of decision making. The parties jointly select one strategy that has the best probability of improving the child's communication and can actually be carried out by the teacher or caregiver (*Example*: Teacher: "I will show Sondra how to ask other children for what she wants, by first saying the name of the child, and then the name of the toy, while the children are playing quietly next to each other.") The fifth and last step involves verification. The teacher or the caregiver implements the plan and collects the data. Periodically the parties reassess and modify the plan as needed. (*Example*: Teacher: "We found that after two weeks of modeling requests 5 to 10 times during playtime each day for Sondra, she increased her use of requests by 25% and reduced her hitting by 15%.")

SLPs who use a consultation model continue to provide some direct intervention so that they may keep abreast of the student's skill development, learning style, interests, strengths, and needs. Borsch and Oaks (1993) reported that the consultation model also is used at the middle school and high school levels, where the SLP works with the classroom teacher to select the best test format for a student, reword worksheets to match a student's language level, or develop materials that may be used in classroom learning stations.

Team Teaching Model

In a *team teaching model*, the classroom teacher and the SLP both teach from their area of expertise. During a science lesson, for example, the classroom teacher focuses on the scientific concepts while the SLP focuses on the new vocabulary. Prior, proper planning must take place for a team teaching model to play out successfully.

The SLP and classroom teacher must decide how they will divide workload responsibilities related to the classroom organization, the type of lesson design, the materials, the behavior management or conflict resolution approach, time management, the materials modifications and/or adaptations needed, the assessment activities, and accountability exercises (e.g., who conducts the parent-teacher conferences). Team teaching may prove to be very time consuming in the early stages. Once the groundwork has been established, however, all parties benefit from providing services to students in the least restrictive environment. Wadle, (1991) provided an account of a successful team teaching model:

> I team-taught a class one period a week with Marty, a seventh and eighth grade social studies teacher. Our experience illustrates the many, often unanticipated, ways that a single program can address the needs of a group of students. Marty was concerned that 'my kids' never expressed any opinions during class discussions. . . . When I considered the three students who were in Marty's class, I was not surprised that they did not venture an opinion. First, their language deficits and limited cultural literacy precluded their being aware of current events. One of Marty's questions concerned the demolition of the Berlin wall. None of my students had any idea where Berlin was, let alone the historical significance of the wall that had divided the east and west portions of the city. Typically, language-learning disabled students do not, or cannot, read "Time" or newspapers and altogether avoid watching national news on TV.
>
> Marty and I planned a year-long program designed to teach students show to state, substantiate, and defend opinions. Students with limited language skills are usually asked lower level questions, which, as classified in Bloom's taxonomy (Bloom, Engelhart, Furst, Hill, & Krathwohl, 1955) test only knowledge or comprehension. Consequently labeled students frequently have little opportunity to answer the type of questions that will be increasingly required in middle and high school. The program, called What's Your Opinion?, helped students develop and practice the language of evaluation as a natural part of successful communication in the classroom. Several opinion questions were presented weekly, one used as a basis for oral discussion and the other requiring a written response.
>
> At first, the questions were general and students did not need to have read widely to 'be smart' to answer them, for example, whether school should be in session year round, or what the best bad-for-you junk food was. Later questions, however, related directly to the seventh-grade social studies syllabus, such as whether we should return land to Native Americans that had been unfairly taken from them in the past. Written answers were graded and counted as a completed assignment, with detailed comments included with every assignment handed back. As the students' skill increased, they were required to use textbooks, the newspaper, Junior Scholastic, and similar sources to gather background and supporting arguments. Cooperative learning groups were frequently used, with labeled students placed in **heterogeneous**, not **homogeneous**, teams. Class sessions were regularly videotaped. . . . Each week after written opinions were completed, six students were chosen by lot. Copies of their opinions were typed, individually framed, mounted, and placed on a bulletin board in the front hall of the school next to their photographs. The camera work was done by three other students who were credited for their photographic talent. During the second semester, the students also created opinion questions for second graders, which provide them an opportunity to practice this meta-linguistic skill of adjusting language for students younger than themselves. It is instructive to read the following guidelines that Marty and I created for the program because they speak so clearly to the shared nature of our collaborative endeavor:
>
> - Regardless of ability, all students will contribute opinions during discussions as well as through written assignments.
> - Both the SLP and the classroom teacher will be supportive and encouraging, even

when neither agrees with the students' responses.

- Teachers will restate or clarify opinions as necessary so that all group members can follow the direction of the discussion.
- Conversations should be as free flowing as possible; strict adherence to "raise your hand before speaking" will not be required.
- All groups will be heterogeneous, and only rarely will cooperative learning groups be formed other than at random.
- When background information is given by one of the teachers, written outlines will be used to limit "lecture time."
- Even when the topic is serious, the tone of the classroom will be as light as possible within the parameters of appropriate classroom behavior.
- Before each completed written assignment is returned, detailed written reactions of the teacher/SLP will be added.
- As much as possible, the opinion question will feature the current week's curriculum topic.
- Each student will be encouraged to use the word-processing program on the classroom computer, the camera, and the videotaping equipment.

As a result of this program, students gained skill in thinking up, formulating, and answering questions that required evaluation, the highest level of thought in Bloom's taxonomy. Students also learned to back up their opinions with cogent reasons and to appreciate the ideas of others, even if they did not agree with them. They learned skills in interviewing and utilizing the word processor and camera as tools. They also discovered ways to find facts as they listened to or read background information, and they gained increased awareness of the larger world around them. Finally, they applied these new skills directly to the seventh-grade social studies curriculum in the presence of their typical classmates. In a pull out program, they would have had little opportunity to do so. (p. 277)

Prevention Model

The *prevention model* is used with students who appear to have learning disabilities. Before IDEA '04, schools had to wait until the student failed before a referral could be made to an IEP team. IDEA '04 facilitated a more proactive approach to see if a student responds to scientifically based, research-based intervention. This proactive concept has been around since the late 1970s, when it was known as "diagnostic teaching" (McCoy, 1995); by the 1990s, it became known as "dynamic assessment" (McCormick, Frome Loeb, & Schiefelbusch, 1997; Merritt & Culatta, 1998; Meyen, Vergason, & Whelan, 1996). Although not specifically mentioned in IDEA '04, the concept is now known as **responsiveness-to-intervention** (RTI).

Boswell (2005) reported that up to 40% of children are in special education because they were not taught how to read. The RTI model is designed to provide children who are at risk for failing in the early grades with scientific research-based intervention as soon as they show signs of academic struggle. Under IDEA '04, school districts may use up to 15% of their Part B funds for early intervention services. The proactive, prevention model is designed to help schools districts differentiate children who simply need high-quality instruction by highly trained educators from those who, despite such instruction, continue to demonstrate underachievement as a result of a disability. The RTI model also may help SLPs differentiate language differences from language disorders among students who are English language learners. Many RTI programs use a three-tiered model such as the one described by Boswell (2005).

- *Tier 1*—Scientifically based instructional practices and behavioral supports are provided for all students, and curriculum-based assessment is used to guide instruction.
- *Tier 2*—Students who do not learn at the rate of their peers receive specialized instruction and/or remediation within the general education classroom.

- *Tier 3*—Students who do not succeed with Tier 2 supports receive a comprehensive evaluation to determine eligibility for special education and related services.

The goal of RTI is to provide differentiated instruction and remedial opportunities in general education. Special education is provided only for those students who require more specialized services.

Cooperative Learning Team Model

Damon and Phelps (1989) defined cooperative learning as a range of team-based learning approaches. During cooperative learning activities, students with varied levels of ability (e.g., a gifted and talented student, two or three students of average ability, and a student with a disability) are divided into small teams. Each heterogeneous team of students is assigned a task, and all of the team members work together to complete that task. The parts of an assigned task often are divided evenly among the members of a team. As described by Meyen, Vergeson, and Whelan (1996), in the cooperative learning model, all team members monitor, assist each other, and provide feedback on one another's work.

Teachers who embrace cooperative learning formats often welcome the SLP into the classroom because the formats rely heavily on verbal language skills. Therefore, it is advantageous to have more than one adult in the room circulating among the small groups as they complete their academic tasks. The SLP who works with students in a cooperative learning classroom has numerous opportunities to infuse oral language goals from each student's IEP into the cooperative learning activities while using materials from the classroom and focusing on curriculum-based educational standards.

Examples of cooperative learning formats described by Kagan (1990) are presented next:

- *Round Robin*: Each student expresses ideas and opinions regarding the assigned task while sitting in small heterogeneous groups. Round Robin is designed to enhance team building and often is used as an activity for getting acquainted.
- *Corners*: Each student moves to a corner of the room that represents a teacher-determined viewpoint. Students discuss within their corner group and then listen to and paraphrase ideas from the other corner groups. This activity is designed to help students see alternative viewpoints and learn how to respect conflicting viewpoints. It also enhances problem-solving approaches to learning.
- *Match Mine*: Students are allowed to use only oral communication as they try to match the arrangement of objects on another student's grid. Match Mine is designed to build vocabulary, oral communication, and pragmatic skills.
- *Numbered Heads Together*: The teacher asks a question and all of the students in the group discuss the answer until they are sure everyone understands it. Then the teacher randomly selects a student from the group to provide the answer. Numbered Heads Together is used as a review activity before an exam or quiz.
- *Color-Coded Co-op Cards*: A flashcard game is used to memorize facts. A group baseline score is recorded and the student team gets points for each additional fact learned by every member of the group. Color-Coded Co-op is used for memorization of facts.
- *Pairs Check*: Students work in pairs within groups of four. Within the **dyad,** one student solves the problem while the other one coaches. After every two problems, they switch roles. Then the two pairs check with each other to see if they achieved the same answers. Pairs Check is used for mass practice.
- *Three-Step Interview*: Students interview each other in pairs. Then they report to the small group what they learned about the other person's information.

Three-Step Interview may be used at the conclusion of a unit.

- *Think-Pair-Share*: When the teacher is using a lecture-listen format, he or she stops every 7 to 10 minutes to ask a reflective question. The students take a moment to answer the question in their heads and then turn to the person next to them and share their answer. Think-Pair-Share is used to enhance inductive reasoning and deductive reasoning.

- *Team Word Web*: Students work together to create a visual map of the main idea or concepts, supporting elements, and bridges representing relationships between the supporting elements. Team Word Web is used for analysis and understanding of multiple relationships.

- *Roundtable*: Each student in the small group answers one question from a set as the list of questions is passed around the group. Roundtable is used to assess prior knowledge, practice, or recall information.

- *Inside-Outside Circle*: Students stand in pairs in two concentric circles. The inside circle faces out and the outside circle faces in. Student use flashcards or respond to teacher questions as they rotate to each new partner. Inside-Outside Circle is used for checking understanding and review.

- *Partners*: Students work in pairs to create or master content. They consult with partners from other teams. Then they share their products with the other students in their small group. Partners is used to enhance mastery of the material and for concept development.

- *Jigsaw*: Each student leaves his or her home group and joins a working group in which he or she explores one aspect of the task with the other group members. Then the students leave their working groups to go back to their home group, where they each report their expert material. Jigsaw is used for the acquisition and presentation of new material.

- *Co-op Co-op*: Students work in groups to produce a product to share with the whole class. Co-op Co-op is used to enhance comprehension of complex material from multiple sources.

Patricia Wildgen, an SLP practicing in Madison, Wisconsin, used a cooperative learning model in a fourth grade that contained four students from her caseload who had oral language goals on their IEPs. She was in the classroom for 45 minutes once a week. She planned the activity and taught it to the whole class. The classroom teacher, who remained in the room during the lesson, was able to learn specific language-enhancing strategies that were modeled; she also facilitated additional cues and prompts within the small groups. Part of every session included dividing the children into small groups and using many of the formats described by Kagan (1990).

Teaming for Reading Model

SLPs often work with children who have oral language disabilities that negatively affect literacy development. In the *teaming for reading* model of service delivery, the SLP teams with other educators for the purpose of developing literacy in school-aged children. The connection between oral and written language is well documented (ASHA, 2001b). Reading development is significantly improved when interventions integrate both the spoken and the written modalities of language. Gillon (2000) reported that collaboration between SLPs and others who have expertise in the development of reading provides greater benefits to students than does traditional speech and language intervention.

The Students Aiming for Achievement in Reading Instruction (SAFARI) program is one such literacy development program. Toennies, Bauman, and Huntenburg (2002) described the SAFARI program as a set-up in which two SLPs team with a reading specialist, a learning disabilities teacher, an occupational therapist, and an educational assistant to provide reading instruction for all children in general education and special education. The program operated Monday through Thursday throughout the academic year. All of the children in first grade were given 30 minutes of language comprehension instruction 4 days per week and 25 minutes of fine motor instruction 1 day per week. This project yielded a coordinated language and reading program for all children. It included a sequential, **multisensory phonics** instruction, activities in **phonological awareness**, instruction in story grammar, vocabulary development, comprehension development, reasoning skill development, letter formation, and fine motor skill development. Each educator involved in the program taught from his or her strength. The SLPs focused on phonological awareness, story grammar, vocabulary building, comprehension, and reasoning skill development. The occupational therapist focused on letter formation and fine motor skill development. The reading specialist and the learning disabilities teacher focused on phonics instruction. As stated in ASHA (2003), the SAFARI program resulted in a more efficient workload strategy. By using this inclusive practice approach, the SLPs had more time to devote to workload aspects of their positions, rather than just dealing with caseloads. They shared intervention responsibilities with an entire team in a more intensive effort.

Shared storybook reading (SSR) is another program format in which SLPs team with other educators for the purpose of developing literacy in school-aged children. As stated by Gormely and Ruhl (2005):

> With only one-quarter the vocabulary of their middle class peers, at-risk students are likely to start school behind and the gap between them and their "normally achieving" peers only grows larger (Hart & Risely, 1995) with the passage of time. Indeed, a particularly strong relationship exists between a child's early vocabulary and their [sic] later literacy success (Catts, Fey, Zhang, & Tomblin, 1999; Snow, Burns, & Griffin, 1998). Young children with poor vocabulary skills are at significant risk for later reading difficulties. Consequently, children with language-related difficul-

ties make up over half the population of students served under IDEA (U.S. Department of Education, 2002). (p. 11)

SSR involves reading a story aloud to children while engaging them in a discussion that is rich in language-enhancing techniques. SSR focuses on teaching the meanings of unfamiliar words, exposing the learners to content that may otherwise be too challenging, providing **decontextualized** experiences, providing repeated exposure to new words, integrating new information with prior knowledge, encouraging interactive dialogue with an adult, encouraging self-expression, and developing listening skills. Gormley and Ruhl (2005) listed six language-enhancing techniques used during SSR. A summary of Gormley and Ruhl's work is provided here:

1. *Modeling*: During SSR, teachers acted as models by using self-talk or "think alouds" while pondering or commenting on the story. They also modeled appropriate language to students with limited experience or language skills by repeating student comments and expanded their utterances.

2. *Praise/encouraging responses*: During SSR, students were encouraged to engage in dialogue about the story and were praised for their efforts. Teachers created a positive, interactive environment by reinforcing children's responses during SSR. The reinforcement increased the likelihood of student responding and lead to more opportunities for vocabulary understanding and use.

3. *Defining*: During SSR, teachers provided explicit definitions of new vocabulary and concepts. In this somewhat more traditional vocabulary instruction method, students were visually presented with target vocabulary (via picture of object) combined with an oral explanation provided by the teacher.

4. *Labeling*: During SSR, teachers supplied names and labels for new vocabulary and concepts. By pointing out specific pictures that represented target vocabulary, teachers provided students with explicit and repeated exposure

to words and ideas that might otherwise go unnoticed.

5. *Follow-up activities*: Following the SSR inter-action, teachers offered students materials and opportunities to help reinforce newly acquired vocabulary. Art activities, flannel board mate-rials, dramatization, and play provided occasions to practice new ideas and concepts within the classroom setting.

6. *Summarizing*: Following SSR, teachers as well as students summarized the story. Summariza-tion required students to use new vocabulary in a meaningful context. It also provided teachers with an opportunity to review vocabulary and concepts, while providing alternate wording to help students with vocabulary understanding. (Gormley & Ruhl, 2005, pp. 11–13)

Pull-Out Program Model

In the classic pull-out model, the SLP removes the child from the general education classroom and works in a separate, isolated environment in either a one-to-one setting or small group setting. The SLP may use materials from the general education curriculum and intertwine the program goals into the activities that focus on curriculum-based con-tent. The SLP also may use specialized materials that focus specifically on the IEP goal. Sessions are held from 1 to 5 days per week, and the amount of time per session may range from 10 to 90 minutes, depending on the specific needs of the child. If the IEP team determines that the pull-out format is the most appropriate model to meet the student's needs, then a rationale statement describing why the student must be removed from the regular education classroom must be included on the student's IEP.

Selecting the Intervention Approach

Each new service delivery format, as described, has inherent strengths and is associated with specific

challenges. The self-contained and the resource room models could arguably be in noncompli-ance with the mandate of providing services in the least restrictive environment. Self-contained, resource room, and pull-out models do not allow opportunities for interactions between students with disabilities and students without disabilities. Those types of interactions are necessary for the social development of both groups. The con-sultation model relies heavily on the SLP's ability to train and supervise others in how to execute clinical methods. Currently, the ASHA does not require specific clinical clock hours in the area of consultation or supervision services. Thus, it is not known how thoroughly graduate schools train such skills. The quality of the consultation will only be as good as the knowledge base of the SLP in the areas of consultation methods and supervision strategies. The team teaching model is time intensive because success relies heavily on collaborative team planning. Time to conduct collaborative planning is hard to find. The cooper-ative learning, teaming for reading, and team teaching models may be efficient only in larger school districts, where several students on one caseload are found in one classroom. Use of this approach may not be possible for the SLP who works in a small, rural district or for the SLP who travels among several schools. The prevention model holds its own unique challenge. In this age of accountability, how do educators document effectiveness if the disability never surfaces as a result of effective prevention efforts?

Each model holds its own promises and pitfalls. It is up to the IEP team to determine the appropriate service delivery model based on the needs of the individual student. Those needs may change dramatically from one school year to the next. Budget planning and personnel time allocations must remain flexible and allow for fluid transitions among service delivery models. In this age of dwindling resources, maintaining flexibility presents its own challenge. Neverthe-less, SLPs and their school systems have found ways to make innovative programs work, as evi-denced by all of the examples provided in this chapter.

Summary

The traditional pull-out remediation approach that was used when school-based SLP services were first introduced in the 1900s still exists today. The evidence-based research indicates that school-based SLPs resort to the traditional pull-out therapeutic approach when they are faced with high caseloads even though researchers have shown that traditional pull-out programs have not worked well (Borsch & Oaks, 1993). New remediation approaches began to evolve in the late 1980s, expanded in the 1990s, and have become more prevalent as a result of the mandates set forth in NCLB and IDEA '04. Other models that have evolved include self-contained classrooms, resource rooms, consultation services, team-teaching, response to intervention, cooperative learning, and teaming for reading.

Questions for Application and Review

1. What are the advantages of the traditional pull-out intervention approach?
2. What are the disadvantages of the traditional pull-out intervention approach?
3. How are the self-contained classroom model and the resource room model alike?
4. How are the self-contained classroom model and the resource room model different?
5. Describe when it would be most advantageous to use a consultation service delivery model.
6. Create a continuum that reflects the most restrictive environment to the least restrictive environment. Place the following intervention approaches along that continuum: self-contained, teaming for reading, resource room, team teaching, cooperative learning, RTI, and consultation model.
7. What are the advantages of a teaming for reading approach to intervention?
8. What are the disadvantages of a teaming for reading approach to intervention?
9. Why has responsiveness to intervention been introduced as a new approach to intervention?
10. Describe the intervention trends for early childhood, elementary, middle school, and high school SLP services.

References

American Speech-Language-Hearing Association. (2000). *IDEA and your caseload: A template for eligibility and dismissal criteria for students ages 3 to 21*. Rockville, MD: Author.

American Speech-Language-Hearing Association. (2001a). *2000 schools survey*. Rockville, MD: Author.

American Speech-Language-Hearing Association. (2001b). *Roles and responsibilities of speech-language pathologists with respect to reading and writing in children and adolescents* [Position statement]. Available at http://www.asha.org/policy

American Speech-Language-Hearing Association. (2002a). *A workload analysis approach for establishing speech-language caseload standards in the schools: Guidelines*. Rockville, MD: Author.

American Speech-Language-Hearing Association. (2002b). *A workload analysis approach for establishing speech-language caseload standards in the schools* [Position statement]. Rockville, MD: Author.

American Speech-Language-Hearing Association. (2002c). *A workload analysis approach for establishing speech-language caseload standards in the schools* [Technical report]. Rockville, MD: Author.

American Speech-Language-Hearing Association (ASHA). (2003). *A workload analysis approach for establishing speech-language caseload standards in the schools: Implementation guide*. Rockville, MD: Author.

Annett, M. (2002). New caseload policy calls for analysis of school clinicians' total workload. *The ASHA Leader, 7*(16), 12–13.

Annett, M. (2003). Looking at total workload. *The ASHA Leader, 8*(7), 1–12.

Annett, M. (2004). Service delivery success. *The ASHA Leader, 9*(4), 1–12.

Bloom, B., Engelhart, M., Furst, E., Hill, W., & Krathwohl, D. (Eds.). (1956). *Taxonomy of educational objectives: The classification of educational goals. Handbook I: Cognitive domain*. New York: David McKay.

Borsch, J., & Oaks, R. (1993). *The collaboration companion*. East Moline, IL: Linguisystems.

Boswell, S. (2005). Prevention model takes off in schools: A new approach for learning disabilities. *The ASHA Leader, 10*(4), 1–21.

Bowen, C. (1998). *PACT: A broad-based approach*. Retrieved January 20, 2005, from http://members.tripod.com/~CarolineBrown/clinphonology.html

Catts, H. W., Fey, M., Zhang, X., & Tomblin, B. (1999). Language bases of reading and reading disabilities: Evidence from a longitudinal investigations. *Scientific Studies of Reading, 3*, 331–361.

Chaney, A., & Burk, T. (1998). *Teaching oral communication in grades K–8*. Needham Heights, MA: Allyn & Bacon.

Chiang, B., & Rylance, B. (2000). *Wisconsin speech-language pathologists' caseloads: Reality and repercussions*. Oshkosh, WI: University of Wisconsin.

Cirrin, F., Bird, A., Biehl, L., Disney, S., Estomin, E., Rudebusch, J., et al. (2003). Speech-language caseloads in the schools: A workload analysis approach to setting caseload standards. *Seminars in Speech and Language, 24*(3), 155–180.

Damon, W., & Phelps, E. (1989). Critical distinctions among three approaches to peer education. *International Journal of Educational Research, 13*, 9–20.

Feeney, T., Riddle, L., & Benedict, L. (2000). *Giving urban children the language to succeed: A consultative-collaborative model*. Rochester, NY: Rochester Hearing and Speech Center.

Gillon, G. T. (2000). The efficacy of phonological awareness intervention. *Language, Speech, and Hearing Services in Schools, 31*, 126–141.

Gormley, S., & Ruhl, K. (2005). Shared storybook reading: Increasing vocabulary skills in an inclusive classroom setting. *Perspectives on School-Based Issues, 6*(1), 11–13.

Hart, B., & Risely, T.R. (1995). *Meaningful differences in the everyday experiences of young American children*. Baltimore: Brookes.

Haynes, W., Moran, M., & Pindzola, R. (1990). *Communication disorders in the classroom*. Dubuque, IA: Kendall Hunt.

Hodson, B. (2007). *Evaluating and enhancing children's phonological systems*. Greenville, SC: Thinking Publications University.

Hodson, B., & Paden, E. (1991). *Targeting intelligible speech* (3rd ed.). Austin, TX: Pro-Ed.

Kagan, S. (1990). The structural approach to cooperative learning. *Educational Leadership, 47*(4), 12–15.

Karr, S., & Schooling, T. (2001, July). *The impact of high caseloads on speech-language pathology services for children in schools*. Written Statement of the American Speech-Language-Hearing Association to the Virginia Board of Education, Richmond, VA.

Kuder, S. (1997). *Language and communication disabilities*. Needham Heights, MA: Allyn & Bacon.

Lowe, R. (1993). *Speech-language pathology & related professions in the schools*. Needham Heights, MA: Allyn & Bacon.

McCormick, L., Frome Loeb, D., & Schiefelbusch, R. (1997). *Supporting children with communication difficulties in inclusive settings: School-based intervention*. Needham Heights, MA: Allyn & Bacon.

McCoy, K. (1995). *Teaching special learners in the general education classroom* (2nd ed.). Denver, CO: Love.

McLearie, E., & Gross, F. P. (1996). *Experimental programs for intensive cycle scheduling of speech and hearing therapy classes*. Columbus, OH: Ohio Department of Education.

Merritt, D., & Culatta, B. (1998). *Language intervention in the classroom*. San Diego, CA: Singular.

Meyen, E., Vergason, G., & Whelan, R. (1996). *Strategies for teaching exceptional children in inclusive settings*. Denver, CO: Love.

Moore, M. (2004). Workload analysis: a winning strategy in the schools. *The ASHA Leader, 9*(11), 1–10.

Neidecker, E., & Blosser, J. (1993). *School programs in speech-language organization and management* (3rd ed.). Englewood Cliffs, NJ: Prentice Hall.

O'Connell, P. (1997). *Speech, language, and hearing programs in schools: A guide for students and practitioners*. Gaithersburg, MD: Aspen.

Oyer, H., Hall, B., Haas, W. (1994). *Speech, language, and hearing disorders: A guide for teachers* (2nd ed.). Needham Heights, MA: Allyn & Bacon.

Paul, R. (1995). *Language disorders from infancy through adolescence: Assessment & intervention*. St. Louis, MO: Mosby.

Peters-Johnson, C. (1996). Action: School services. *Language, Speech, and Hearing Services in Schools, 27*, 185–186.

Peters-Johnson, C. (1998). Professional practices perspective on caseloads in schools. *Asha Magazine, 12*, 5.

Simons, C. (1991). *Communication skills and classroom success*. Eau Claire, WI: Thinking Publications.

Snow, C. E., Burns, M. S., Griffin, P. (Eds.). (1998). *Preventing reading difficulties in young children*. Washington, DC: National Academy Press.

Taylor, J. (1992). *Speech-language pathology services in the schools* (2nd ed.). Needham Heights, MA: Allyn & Bacon.

Toennies, J., Bauman, C., Huntenburg, S. (2002). SAFARI: An alternative reading and language program. *Perspectives on School-Based Issues, 3*(1), 12–14.

U.S. Department of Education. (2002). *Twenty-fourth annual report to Congress on the implementation of the Individuals with Disabilities Education Act.* Washington, DC: Author.

Villa, R., & Thousand, J. (1995). *Creating an inclusive school.* Alexandria, VA: Association for Supervision and Curriculum Development.

Wadle, S. (1991). Clinical exchange: Why speech-language clinicians should be in the classroom. *Language, Speech and Hearing Services in Schools, 22*(3), 277.

Whitmire, K. (2003, July). *Workload and caseload: Getting into balance.* Presentation at the annual convention of the American Speech-Language Hearing Association Conference, Anaheim, CA.

Whitmire, K., & Dublinske, S. (2003). Speech-language caseloads in the schools: A workload analysis approach to setting caseload standards. *Seminars in Speech and Language, 24*(3), 147–154.

Whitmire, K., Karr, S., & Mullen., R. (2000). Action: School services. *Language, Speech, and Hearing Service in Schools, 31,* 402–406.

Chapter 5

EVIDENCE-BASED PRACTICE

RELATED VOCABULARY

baseline   the data collected before an intervention is introduced.

baseline risk   The risk that an event will occur without active treatment or intervention.

bias   The alteration in outcome for a study or its findings that can be attributed to the way(s) in which the study is conducted.

blinding/blinded   Referring to a study in which all of the people involved are unaware of which treatment group each participant was assigned to until the results have been interpreted.

controlled clinical trial   A trial in which participants are assigned to two or more different treatment groups.

controls/control subjects   The participants in a comparison group who receive either a placebo, no treatment, or a standard treatment.

cost-benefit analysis   An analytical method that converts effects into the same monetary terms as those for the costs and compares them.

intention to treat (ITT) analysis Analysis of data for all participants based on the group to which they were randomized and not based on the actual treatment they received.

randomized controlled trial A clinical trial in which participants are randomly assigned to two or more groups, with one group receiving an intervention that is being tested and the other group receiving an alternative treatment or placebo.

regression analysis An analytical method of finding the "best" mathematical model to describe or predict the dependent variable as a function of the independent variable(s).

significant Statistically significant at the 5% level. This is the same as a 95% confidence interval not including the value corresponding to no effect.

validity The property of a study or its findings for which the results are unbiased and provide an accurate estimate of the effect that is being measured.

Introduction

The movement for evidence-based practice began in the field of medicine during the 1990s, when Dr. Gordon Guyatt of McMaster University in Hamilton, Ontario introduced the concept as "scientific medicine." His colleagues, however, were offended by the term because they believed it denigrated their professional expertise. In response to this negative reaction, Guyatt renamed the concept "evidence-based medicine," a term his colleagues agreed was more appropriate. Guyatt's newly created phrase, *evidence-based*, mirrored the work of the Cochrane Collaboration, a group of researchers, physicians, and allied health professionals whose goal was to systematically gather and evaluate research related to medical treatments.

The Cochrane Collaboration began its work in 1993 and gained international notoriety in 2005 when its findings showed that there was no credible evidence that vaccinations were the cause of autism spectrum disorders (ASDs). The Cochrane Collaboration based on its review of 139 studies (Gorman, 2007). Guyatt and a colleague, David Sackett, took the work of the Cochrane Collaboration one step further and advocated not only that physicians use medical practices that have a scientific base but that the evidence must be "credible" based on a ranking system. The mandate for evidence-based practice in public schools was strengthened when the No Child Left Behind Act (NCLB) was signed into law in 2002. The NCLB Statement of Purpose proclaimed "school wide reform and ensuring the access of children to effective, scientifically based instructional strategies and challenging academic content" [Sec. 1001 (9)].

"Credible Evidence" and "Scientifically Based": What Do These Terms Mean?

The American Speech-Language-Hearing Association (ASHA, 2006) reported that the U.S. Department of Education Office of Special Education formed a National Research Council (NRC) in 2001. The purpose of the NRC was to create a framework for evaluating the scientific evidence regarding the effectiveness of educational intervention for young children with ASDs. The NRC established guidelines for evaluating the quality of the scientific evidence based on three criteria. These criteria, summarized next, represent the major issues that peer reviewers consider when judging evidence for publications in professional journals.

1. Threats to internal **validity**
   - Does the study include a group of **control subjects (controls)** so that the effects of maturation can be determined?
   - Are the pretest and posttest measures conducted by different persons from those who delivered the treatment?
   - Are the gains merely the result of a statistical artifact (e.g., **regression analysis**?
2. Threats to external validity
   - Were the participants randomly selected or assigned?
   - Is the sample size too small?
   - Is the sample size too large?
   - Were the populations well defined?
3. Generalization
   - Are the treatment outcomes likely outside of the experimental environment? That is, can they be generalized?
   - Are the treatment outcomes functional?

To demonstrate the importance of internal validity, external validity, and generalization, the following Song-and-Dance Therapy example is offered:

Mr. Song-and-Dance claimed that articulation errors can be eliminated by enrolling young children in his private Song-and-Dance Therapy program. His theory is that children who engage in fun, daily gross motor exercise while singing songs develop precise articulation skills. He convinced the local school board to conduct an experiment. When each child in the district reached the age of 4 years, Mr. Song-and-Dance administered an articulation test and collected **baseline** data related to articulation. These data revealed that 60% of the children exhibited articulation errors. Then the children were enrolled in the Song-and-Dance program in lieu of kindergarten. When each child reached the age of 6, the same articulation test was administered by the same dance instructor. The posttest data revealed that only 25% of the children exhibited articulation errors. All of the school board members were very impressed and ready to eliminate all individualized articulation remediation and replace it with the Song-and-Dance Therapy program, because it was so much cheaper and appeared to be very effective. The board members were especially impressed that 35% of the children improved in their articulation skills, as indicated by the data that Mr. Song-and-Dance had provided.

Threats to Internal Validity

In the foregoing example, what the school board did not know is that "Shriberg (1997), in summarizing his previous studies on speech normalization, reported that approximately 75% of children with speech delay normalize their speech errors by age 6" (Kamhi, 2006, p. 273). The conducted by Mr. Song-and-Dance did not include a control group. Thus, there was no way to guarantee that the reduction in articulation errors was not the result of maturation (**baseline risk**). Another problem was that Mr. Song-and-Dance conducted all the testing himself, and his criteria drifted. He had a vested interest in judging close approximations as errors in the pretest and judging close approximation errors as acceptable in the posttest. A third problem arose when the same test was used for both the pretest and posttest. Without a control group, it couldnot be determined whether or not the children achiev-ed better scores simply because they became better test takers on a measure they had seen before.

Threat to External Validity

The sample size that Mr. Song and Dance used in his study was too big and not well defined. It included *all* of the children in the school district, resulting in a regression toward the mean. In such samples, the children who previously scored in the upper and lower ends of the range will get better or worse just by virtue of taking the test a second time. Instead, a subset of children should have been randomly selected and randomly assigned to either a control group or an experimental group.

Generalization

A final big problem is that the Song-and-Dance remediation program is not at all functional. All other aspects of the kindergarten curriculum were abandoned; none of the children made adequate yearly progress; and the school district faced an "At Risk" status with possible sanctions as specified under NCLB.

Criteria for Evaluating the Quality of the Reasoning

In addition to considering the three major criteria just discussed, peer reviewers historically have critically evaluated the reasoning of an author when a study is submitted to a professional journal for publication. Paul and Elder (2007) documented eight characteristics that peer reviewers consider:

1. *Purpose*: Is the purpose clear and understandable?

2. *Question*: Does the question relate to the purpose, and is it unbiased?
3. *Information*: Is a knowledge base provided that supports the purpose and question?
4. *Concepts*: Does the author provide justification through a literature review?
5. *Assumptions*: Does the author make distinctions between facts and assumptions?
6. *Inferences*: Does the author justify conclusions with logical connections?
7. *Point of view*: Does the author remain objective and present all possible sides of the issue or differing points of view?
8. *Implications*: Does the author provide a logical link between facts and identified implications?

Ranking the Quality of the Evidence

The evidence-based practice movement challenged professionals to take the process of critical peer review one step farther. Looking for threats to internal and external validity, judging generalization, and evaluating the purpose, question, information, concepts, assumptions, inferences, point of view and implications of a body of work were not sufficient in the eyes of the evidence-based practice advocates. The movement demanded a specific definition of the term *credible* based on a ranking system and judging the professional work on the basis of the level of evidence it provided. In 2007 the ASHA considered a system for evaluating and ranking evidence; this system was developed by the U.S. Preventive Task Force in 1989. The system is shown in Table 5–1.

ASHA Initiative

In response to the evidence-based practice movement, the ASHA established the National Center for Evidence-Based Practice in Communication Disorders (N-CEP) for the purpose of writing guidelines for the Association. The N-CEP adopted an internationally accepted instrument, the Appraisal

Table 5–1. Evaluating and Ranking Research Evidence

Quality	Designation Criterion/Criteria
Level I	Evidence from at least one well-conducted **randomized** clinical trial
Level II–1	Evidence from one well-conducted study **with controls** but **without randomization**
Level II–2	Evidence from one well-designed **cohort** or **case-control study**, preferably from **independent researchers**
Level II–3	Evidence from **multiple** time-series **single-subject investigations** or **dramatic results from noncontrolled experiments**
Level III	**Opinions of authorities**, descriptive studies, case studies, reports of expert committees

Grade	Recommendation	Designation Criterion
A	Good evidence for inclusion	**Good peer-review evidence** supporting consideration of use for intervention
B	Fair evidence for inclusion	**Fair peer-review evidence** supporting consideration of use for intervention
C	Insufficient evidence	**Insufficient peer-review evidence**, although recommendations for use are possible on other grounds
D	Fair evidence of exclusion	**Fair peer-review evidence** showing the **intervention should be excluded** from consideration of use
E	Good evidence of exclusion	**Good peer-review evidence** showing the **intervention should be excluded** from consideration of use

Source: United States Preventive Services Task Force (1989).

of Guidelines for Research and Evaluation (AGREE) (AGREE Collaboration, 2001), as a framework for assessing the quality of clinical practice guidelines. The AGREE instrument is designed to help the ASHA N-CEP in meeting the following goals:

- Identify or avoid potential **bias**
- Ensure that recommendations are internally valid
- Ensure that recommendations are externally valid
- Ensure that guidelines are feasible for practice
- Assess the potential for benefit and for harm
- Assess the **cost-benefit analysis**
- Assess the practical issues
- Assess the quality of reporting
- Assess the predicted validity

The AGREE introduction proclaimed: "The AGREE was developed through discussion between researchers from several countries who have extensive experience and knowledge of clinical guidelines. Thus, the AGREE instrument should be perceived as reflecting the current state of knowledge in the field" (AGREE Collaboration, 2001, p. 2). Most of the criteria contained in the AGREE instrument are based on theoretical assumptions, rather than on empirical evidence. The AGREE instrument does not assess the impact of a guideline on outcomes for patients, clients, or students.

ASHA Framework for Assessing Levels of Evidence

The AGREE instrument is useful for evaluation of professional guidelines. Another framework was needed, however, to evaluate clinical practice. Thus, the N-CEP collaborated with ASHA's Advisory Committee on Evidence-Based Practice (ACEBP) to create a framework for evaluating levels of evidence of clinical practice. When the ACEBP was created in 2005, its mission was to review all of the different systems that have been created to evaluate levels of evidence, and then to find the one that best fits the needs of the profession. However, the ACEPB discovered two major problems with the existing systems. First, many systems did not use objective criteria to define high- and low-quality studies. Second, most levels of evidence systems were based on a medical model that did not consider single-subject design as credible evidence. Accordingly, the ACEPB created a ranking system unique to clinical practice in the field of communication disorders and sciences. The ACEBP relied heavily on the work of Robey (2004) and created a four-step framework, described next.

Step One

The first step of ASHA's level of evidence system addressed one of the major problems that many other existing systems ignored: appraising the quality of the study using objective criteria. ACEBP created eight criteria for quality appraisal of individual studies. Each criterion lists a hierarchy of quality. For example, under the criteria of study design, the use of a **controlled clinical trial** would yield the highest quality, whereas the use of a case series case would yield the lowest quality. The eight criteria created by the ACEBP were as follows:

- The quality of the study design
- **Blinding**
- Sampling
- Subject selection process

- Outcomes
- Significance
- Precision
- **Intention to treat analysis**

Step Two

The study is identified within a continuum that ranges across four possibilities:

1. Exploratory
2. Efficacy
3. Effectiveness
4. Cost/benefit

The uniqueness of the framework is reflected in this step because the ASHA N-CEP and ACEBP recognized that a single-subject design study may yield the best evidence for a particular research question.

Step Three

The quality of the study is assessed. It is judged within the point at which it falls on the continuum reflected in Step Two.

Step Four

A table that summarizes the evidence related to a specific clinical question is created. This overview of the evidence helps identify which areas of clinical practice already show a sufficient level of evidence, which require more clinical research, and which lead to a new research question.

"Evidence Based" Is More Than Literature Reviews

Justice and Fey (2004) explained that application of evidence-based practice by the school-based speech-language pathologist (SLP) involves more than simply doing a literature review and judging the quality of the evidence. Clinical decisions involve consideration of multiple factors. Justice and Fey identified the primary factors as the SLP's clinical expertise; his or her substantive theoretical knowledge; and the preferences voiced by the student or the family. Other factors that should be considered include effectiveness in the least restrictive environment; effectiveness using curriculum-based intervention; outcomes from the evaluation process that are unique to the student; recommendations from the other members of the individualized education program (IEP) team; the individual's unique needs for achieving a free and appropriate public education; accommodations necessary to participate in statewide and district-wide testing; cultural factors; and the student's needs for achieving transition goals, if applicable.

When Is It Advantageous to Examine Levels of Evidence?

Gillam and Gillam (2006) pointed out that deciding on a course of intervention is facilitated when seven characteristics are present:

1. The results of well-designed studies support the intervention program that the SLP, parents, and other IEP team members have agreed on.
2. The local education agency (LEA) representative is willing to commit resources toward it.
3. The IEP builds on the child's strengths, interests, and learning style.
4. The goals address the child's challenges.
5. The goals are curriculum based.
6. The SLP and other team members are well trained to execute the program.
7. The program is executed in the least restrictive environment that is appropriate for the child.

As might be expected, the relationship among all of these factors is not always harmonious. Gillam and Gillam provided the following example.

The parents of a child with a communication disorder demanded that the school district's language and reading program be replaced with a *Fast ForWord-L* program. This scenario demonstrated a situation in which the IEP team used a methodical procedure for decision-making purposes. Gillam and Gillam (2006) recommended framing the clinical question so that it included four important parts:

- The population (P)
- The investigative aspect (I)
- The control (C)
- The objective measure (O)

"In intervention with (P) primary-grade children with language-based learning disabilities, does (I) *Fast ForWord-L* or (C) traditional language intervention and reading instruction result in the greater improvement on (O) measures of language and reading?" (Gillam & Gillam, p. 309).

In this example, the literature shows that three studies were judged to be Level 1 quality (Cohen et al., 2005; Pokorni, Worthington, & Jamison, 2004; Rouse & Kruger, 2004), and another supportive study was judged to be Level 2 quality (Hook, Macaruso, & Jones, 2001). These four studies indicated that *Fast ForWord-L* did not yield better language or reading outcomes than other computer-assisted instruction or reading and language instruction that was being provided. Thus, the school district had ample evidence to support the decision to deny the parents request to replace the current program with the *Fast ForWord-L* program. This example illustrates the process that Gillam and Gillam adapted from the work of Porzsolt and colleagues (2003). They encouraged school-based SLPs to use this process to create their own evidence base for preferred practice patterns where no other evidence exists. The recommended seven-step process follows:

Step 1: Create a general or specific clinical question.

Step 2: Find external evidence that pertains to the question.

Step 3: Determine the level of evidence that the study represents and critically evaluate the study.

Step 4: Evaluate the internal evidence related to the student-parent factors.

Step 5: Evaluate the internal evidence related to clinician-agency factors.

Step 6: Make a decision by integrating the evidence.

Step 7: Evaluate the outcomes of the decision.

Challenges

School-based SLPs face at least two major challenges when charged with creating their own evidence base for preferred practice patterns where no other evidence exists. The first major challenge is the time necessary to complete the task. Gillam and Gillam (2006) documented that it takes the Scottish Intercollegiate Guidelines Network approximately two years to go through a series of 50 steps to determine the quality of evidence related to a specific topic. If it takes a team of 15 to 20 persons with the assistance of professional librarians and biostatisticians working full time for two years to complete this process, then how realistic is it to ask school-based SLPs to create their own evidence when such activities are not identified in the SLP's workload?

The second major challenge facing the school-based SLP is the unique characteristics of each student on his or her caseload. The outcomes of studies designed for homogeneous groups may not be applicable to the program in question. In a student profile taken from an actual school-based SLP's caseload, for example, the student was bilingual, deaf, and visually impaired and had an ASD. How would this student fit into the evidence-based practice research related to intervention efficacy?

The quality of the outcome may be only as good as the quality of the question posed. This point is admirably illustrated by Carney and Moeller (1998): " . . . treatment efficacy cannot and should not be considered independently of the goals of treatment for children with hearing loss. These goals may be as diverse and as heterogeneous as the population of children" (p. S61).

State of the Art

Tables 5–2 to 5–10 summarize the professional literature of studies that have been peer-reviewed and published in professional journals. The peer reviews were based on critical analysis of the following 11 characteristics:

- Threats to internal validity
- Threats to external validity
- Generalization
- Evaluation of the purpose
- The question
- The information
- The concepts
- The assumptions
- The inferences
- The point of view
- The implications

Of note, these studies have not yet been ranked on the recommended levels of evidence set forth by the U.S. Preventive Services Task Force (1989). That is the next step necessary to achieve the level of scientific rigor advocated by the N-CEP and ACEBP.

The N-CEP completed its first evidence-based systematic review (EBSR) of aphasia intervention approaches in 2007. As additional reviews are conducted, findings will be included in the ASHA Practice Policy, available at www.asha.org/policy as a new type of technical report. Until N-CEP completes analysis of all types of clinical approaches, the information in the accompanying tables may be useful to the SLP who is asked to show the evidence base of a proposed remediation approach. If a parent opposes the recommended approach and advocates for a different approach, then it is necessary for all parties involved to pursue the analysis described by Gillam and Gillam (2006). The Web-based resources presented in Appendix 5–1 may be of value if such an analysis is required.

Specific Evidence of What Works in Speech-Language Intervention

Phonology Intervention

Background

General Gierut (2007) documented that deficits in the production of speech sounds can result from physical, organic, or functional causes and are the most prevalent communication disability diagnosed in preschool- and school-aged children. Approximately 10% of this population exhibit phonological disorders. Children with phonological disorders are at risk for reading and writing disabilities (Gierut, 2007). If unresolved, phonological disorders may inhibit development of the affected person's social, academic, and vocational abilities.

General Recommendations

Clinical evidence has documented that children benefit from services provided by an SLP. The goal of intervention is to increase the accuracy and use of speech sounds to achieve maximum intelligibility. According to the National Outcomes Measurement System (NOMS) conducted by the ASHA, 70% of preschool children who received phonological treatment demonstrated increased intelligibility and communication functioning. The amount of intervention plays a **significant** role in the outcome. The 70% of the children in this population who achieved intelligible speech received roughly twice as much intervention as that provided for the 30% whose speech remained unintelligible (ASHA, 2003). Several different intervention approaches have been shown to be efficacious. Table 5–2 presents the supportive evidence for those approaches typically used by school-based SLPs. No single approach is endorsed over another.

Language Intervention

Background

Goldstein and Prelock (2007) documented that language delays and disorders in children may result from head injury, hearing loss, toxins, diseases, or congenital syndromes. Approximately 7% of preschool and school-age children exhibit disabilities in understanding and/or using spoken language. SLPs play an important role in providing optimal treatment for children with language disabilities.

General Recommendations

According to the NOMS, 70% of preschool children who received language intervention from an SLP achieved gains on functional communication measures. The amount of intervention plays a significant role in the outcome. Children who made gains received approximately twice as much intervention as that provided for the children who did not show functional improvement (ASHA, 2002b).

Table 5–2. Evidence of What Works: Phonology Intervention

Intervention Perspective	Supportive Evidence
Normative approach—A developmental approach introducing the target sounds following the typical developmental sequence, with nasals, stops, and glides acquired early and fricatives, affricates, and consonant clusters acquired later	Gillon, 2005 Howell & Dean, 1994 Metsala & Walley, 1998 Nittrouer, 2002 Oller, 1978 Velleman & Vihman, 2002 Vihman, 2004 Walley, Metsala, & Garlock, 2003

continues

Table 5–2. *continued*

Intervention Perspective	Supportive Evidence
Traditional motor approach—Begins with discrimination training followed by production of the sound in isolation, nonsense syllables, words, structured phrases, sentences, and then spontaneous speech; a high criteria (e.g., 85% correct production) must be achieved before the next level of difficulty is introduced	Bernthal & Bankson, 2004 Van Riper & Emerick, 1984
Language-based approach combined with direct approach—Views phonology as an integral and inseparable part of the language constellation; uses illustrated storybooks as the principal remediation context to teach sound discrimination, sound production, prosody, and phonological awareness; provides more frequent production cues for children with motor speech disorders such as developmental apraxia; *use this approach in conjunction with approaches that target speech production directly*	Camarata, 1993 Norris & Hoffman, 2005 Tyler, Lewis, Haskill, & Tolbert, 2002 Tyler & Sandoval, 1994
Cycles approach—Combines elements of traditional motor placement with a additional perceptual component, an efficient goal attack strategy, and phonological assessment; treatment selection is based on the normative perspective, with an understanding that acquisition is gradual; no predetermined criterion for phoneme mastery	Hodson & Padden, 1991 Lof & Watson, 2005
Complexity approach—Uses more complex linguistic input promote the greatest change in a child's overall sound system; targeting difficult sounds leads to better generalization of untreated sounds that does targeting easier sounds first (e.g., target /v/ and get spontaneous generalization of /f/); targeting affricates improves fricatives; targeting clusters improves singletons, targeting fricatives improves stops, targeting nonstimulable sounds improves stimulable sounds, and targeting voiced stops improves voiceless stops	Gierut, 2001, 2005 Miccio & Ingrisano, 2000 Weston & Bain, 2003 Williams, 2005
Broad-based approach—A flexible theoretical orientation; eclectic approach; uses whatever works for the individual child, synthesizing bits and pieces from multiple perspectives; adapts in accordance with the individual student's needs	Gersten & Brengelman, 1996 Kamhi, 1994, 1999, 2006
Structured home carryover program coupled with school services—Data from the ASHA National Outcomes Measurement System (NOMS) have shown that the proportion of children making significant gains in speech is more than doubled when the children participate in a structured home program	ASHA, 2002b
Individual versus group intervention—More intervention time in individual sessions results in more functional gains	ASHA, 2002b
Transition remediation approach based on progress—Begin with individualized, short, intensive sessions 4 to 5 times per week and then decrease the frequency to once a week, coupled with a home carryover program as progress is made	Gillam et al., 2005 Jacoby, Lee, Kummer, Levin & Creghead, 2002 Tylor, 2005

Roth and Paul (2007) advocated for the use of a continuum of naturalness based on the client's individual needs:

> Research evidence supports the use of both naturalistic and structured intervention approaches with a broad range and severity of speech, language, and communication disorders for children (e.g., Conture, 1996; Geirut, 1998; Hemmeter, Ault, Collins & Meyer, 1996; Kim, Yang, & Hwang, 2001; Kouri, 2005; Swanson, Fey, Mills, & Hood, 2005) and adults (Conture, 1996; Holland, Fromm, DeRuyter & Stein, 1996; Robey, 1998; Ramig & Verdolini, 1998). (p. 171)

Several different remediation approaches have been shown to be efficacious. Studies have confirmed the advantage of beginning intervention as early as possible (McLean & Woods Cripe, 1997).

Table 5–3 presents sources for the supportive evidence for those clinical approaches that typically are used by school-based SLPs. No single approach is endorsed over another.

Social Aspects of Communication in Autism Spectrum Disorders

Background

ASDs include Asperger syndrome, pervasive developmental disorder, Rett Syndrome and childhood disintegrative disorders. Persons with these disorders often exhibit impairments in speech, language, social, or cognitive abilities. Clinical evidence shows that children and adults who receive intervention from an SLP make significant gains, especially if the intervention begins at an early age (Prelock,

Table 5–3. Evidence of What Works: Language

Intervention Perspective	Supportive Evidence
Indirect language stimulation/ expansions—The SLP reformulates what the child said into an expanded, grammatically complete sentence. (*Example:* Child: "That a truck." SLP: "Oh! That's a big red truck with black wheels.")	Law, Garrett, & Nye, 2004 Roth & Paul, 2007
Focused language stimulation—The SLP manipulates the environment to evoke the child's spontaneous production of a specific linguistic target using strategies such as false assertions, feigned misunderstandings, forced choices, contingent query, violation of routines, and/or withholding objects or turns. The SLP also provides frequent models in meaningful, highly functional contexts.	Weismer & Robertson, 2006 Fey, Cleave, & Long, 1997 Owens, 2004 Paul, 2007
Clinician-directed approach—The SLP controls all aspects of the intervention (e.g., determining goals, selecting materials, controlling the type and frequency of reinforcement, designing the order of the activities, identifying the desired responses). The SLP uses specific clinical techniques such as cues, fading cues as specific target criteria are met, verbal prompts, shaping, and delayed imitation.	Fey, Cleave, & Long, 1997 Roth & Worthington, 2005 Skinner, 1957
Client-centered approach—Remediation is conducted in authentic settings; newly learned behaviors are evoked and/or reinforced by using expansions, extensions, and/or recasts in the context of familiar experiences and activities with supportive communication partners.	Fey, 1986

continues

Table 5–3. *continued*

Intervention Perspective	Supportive Evidence
Facilitative play approach—The SLP models target language forms and functions using self-talk and/or parallel talk during client-centered activities in authentic settings. The child's interest is maintained by using high-interest, developmentally appropriate activities.	Owens, 2004 Paul, 2007
Parent-directed—The SLP models specific techniques while interacting with the child; the parent observes; parent's questions are answered; then the SLP observes the parent use the techniques while the SLP observes; the SLP provides specific positive and/or corrective feedback to the parent; a home carryover program is established.	Fey et al., 1997
Model imitation/modeling plus evoked production—The SLP provides a model of the target and the child imitates it. Specific verbal praise and corrective feedback are provided. Edible, tangible, social, and/or natural reinforcements may or may not be provided.	Ellis Weismer & Murray-Branch, 1989
Recast—The SLP expands the child's utterance into a different sentence type. (*Example:* Child: "That a truck." SLP: "Is that a truck?")	Fey, Cleave, & Long, 1997 Nelson, Camarata, Welsh, Butkovsky & Camarata, 1996
Target-specific recast—The SLP expands the child's utterance and includes a specific language target using emphatic stress. (*Example:* Child: "That a truck." SLP: "That *is* a big truck.")	Fey, Cleave, & Long, 1997
Functional approach—The SLP offers linguistic support and scaffolding while the child or adolescent engages in activities of daily living.	Roth & Paul, 2007
Hybrid approach—The SLP uses activities that are natural; controls the environment; and incorporates a variety of techniques based on the individual student's learning style to maximize learning and generalization.	Fey, 1986
Milieu teaching—The SLP uses ongoing activities as the basis for intervention and incorporates the operant principles of imitation, modeling, and reinforcement into natural settings.	Hart & Risley, 1975 Warren & Kaiser, 1986 Rogers-Warren & Warren, 1980 Warren, 1991
Script—The SLP teaches target behaviors within a familiar routine that has a specific sequence (e g., ordering a pizza, withdrawing money from a savings account, washing dishes). Once the script is learned, the SLP violates the routine (i.e., not removing the wrap before cooking a food item) as a way to evoke more complex language. The script may also be used to teach time concepts and tense markers (e.g., before, after, yesterday, tomorrow).	Olswang & Bain, 1991 Weismer & Evans, 2002
Interrupted-behavior chain strategy—The SLP introduces a new intervention target into a script that has been well learned in an authentic context. The SLP uses model imitation, verbal prompts, specific verbal praise, and specific corrective feedback	Caro & Snell, 1989
Target drill, drill play—The SLP uses visual cues such as flashcards or photographs that depict a specific linguistic target. The child verbalizes the target in short, rapid, multiple trials. (*Example for pronoun use:* Child: "He is running. She is eating. They are singing.")	Fey, 1986 Paul, 2007 Roth & Worthington, 2005

2007). The current estimated prevalence for ASD in the United States is 34 per 10,000 (Yeargin-Allsopp et al., 2003). The National Institutes of Health (2001) reported that approximately 1 of every 250 births are affected by ASDs. According to the National Outcomes Measurement System (NOMS) conducted by ASHA (2002b), two thirds of preschoolers with ASD achieve gains in functional communication, spoken language, and social use of language after intervention provided by an SLP.

General Recommendations

A comprehensive study conducted by the NRC (2001) documents that children with ASD who participate in intensive intervention beginning at the age of 3 years have a significantly better outcome than that in children beginning intervention after age 5. Children with ASD require intensive, instructional programming a minimum of 5 hours per day, 5 days per week. They require instructional opportunities that are organized in a series of brief time intervals and include systematically planned, developmentally appropriate learning activities with a sufficient amount of adult attention. Children with ASD require individualized attention on a daily basis. A student-to-staff ratio of no more than two young children with ASD per adult in the classroom are recommended. Children with ASD should receive programming that allows for: functional, spontaneous communication; social interaction in various settings; facilitation of play skills with peers; generalization of newly learned skills in natural contexts; positive behavioral support; and functional academic skill development.

Table 5-4 provides the supportive evidence for those clinical approaches that typically are used by school-based SLPs. No single approach is endorsed over another.

Table 5–4. Evidence of What Works: Social Communication Intervention

Intervention Perspective	Supportive Evidence
Conversational group therapy approach—Group members engage in conversations while the SLP provides attending cues, facilitative questions, negotiations, verbal praise for spontaneous production of targets, modeling, mediating, prompting, gate-keeping, and summarizing.	Ewing, 1999 Roth & Paul, 2007
Conversational coaching—The SLP stimulates conversational interaction in a structured context by providing a model of short, meaningful utterances as a written script that the client imitates. The topic is selected based on the client's interests. The client reads the script aloud one sentence at a time using gestures, if necessary, to convey meaning. The client is videotaped, and the tape is replayed to an unfamiliar listener. The listener rates his or her ability to understand what the client said. The three evaluate the video to determine the most and least helpful strategies. The process is repeated multiple times.	Holland, 1995
Collaborative model—The SLP establishes partnerships with families. The family defines its level of involvement. The SLP provides the family with information and teaches the family interaction skills, behavioral management skills, and strategies to enhance language development.	National Research Council, 2001

continues

Table 5-4. *continued*

Intervention Perspective	Supportive Evidence
Co-model—The SLP and the family play complementary roles in developing goals and executing an intervention plan.	Marcus, Kunce, & Schopler, 2005
Behavioral model—Family members learn and apply specific behavior-shaping strategies.	Marcus, Kunce, & Schopler, 2005
Cognitive approach—Family members learn problem-solving strategies, cognitive restructuring, and how to set realistic expectations.	Marcus, Kunce, & Schopler, 2005
Emotional support—Professionals provide empathetic listening and teach problem-solving strategies for concerns that the family has identified.	Marcus, Kunce, & Schopler, 2005
Advocacy training—Professionals assist families in learning how to advocate for services and system changes. The SLP, intervention team, professionals, and/or family promote self-determination in children with ASDs.	Marcus, Kunce, & Schopler, 2005 Westling & Fox, 2000 Baker, Horner, Suppington & Ard, 2000
Natural language paradigm—An ecological approach in which communication competence is fostered in natural settings.	Koegel, O'Dell, & Koegel, 1987
Incidental teaching—Language skills of labeling and describing are learned in naturally occurring activities during adult-child interactions.	Hart, 1985 McGee, Krantz, & McClannahan, 1985 McGee, Morrier, & Daly, 1999
Time delay, milieu intervention—The SLP, intervention team, educators, professionals, and/or family use ongoing activities as the basis for intervention and incorporates the operant principles of imitation, modeling, and reinforcement into natural settings.	Charlop, Schreibman, & Thibodeau, 1985 Hwang & Hughes, 2000b Kaiser, 1993 Kaiser, Yoder, & Keetz, 1992
Pivotal response training—The SLP, intervention team, educators, professionals, and/or family allow choice over the nature of the interaction and materials used in a natural context and reinforce the attempt to respond for the child with an ASD.	Koegel, 1995 Koegel, Camarata, Koegel, Ben-Tall, & Smith, 1998 Whalon & Schreibman, 2003
Developmental strategies—The SLP, intervention team, educators, professionals, and/or parents teach language comprehension and production based on a model of typical development and sequence.	Aldred, Greer, & Adams, 2004 Hwang & Hughes, 2000b Lewy & Dawson, 1992 Mahoney & Perales, 2005 Rogers & Lewis, 1989 Greenspan & Wieder, 1997 Prizant & Wetherby, 1998
Positive behavior support—The SLP, intervention team, educators, and/or family directly target the relationship between challenging behavior and communication. The scientific practice of applied behavior analysis is incorporated into a person-centered, comprehensive program with a focus on intervention in the natural context to use prevention strategies, foster replacement skills, and respond in a positive manner.	Horner, Albin, Sprague, & Todd, 2000

Table 5–4. *continued*

Intervention Perspective	Supportive Evidence
Teach functional equivalents—The SLP, intervention team, and/or family teach the child with an ASD communication functions (e.g., to request objects, request assistance, express frustration, or seek attention) to replace undesirable behaviors.	Carr et al., 2002 Durand & Carr, 1991, 1992 Horner, Day, Sprague, O'Brian, & Heathfield, 1991 Horner, Albin, Sprague, & Todd, 2000 Lalli, Casey, & Kates, 1995
Augmentative-assistive technology and methods—The SLP, intervention team, educators, and/or family teach the child with an ASD to use alternative communication modalities to engage in social interactions.	Barrera, Lobatas-Barrera, Sulzer-Azaroff, 1980 Barrera & Sulzer-Azaroff, 1983 Bopp, Brown, & Mirenda, 2004 Brady, 2000 Frea, Arnold, & Vittimberga, 2001 Ganz & Simpson, 2004 Garrison-Harrell, Kamps, & Kravits, 1997 Layton, 1988 Light, Roberts, DiMarco, & Greiner, 1998 Mirenda, 1997a, 1997b , 2003 Peterson, Bonday, Vincent, & Finnegan, 1995 Shane & Simmons, 2001 Wendt, Schlosser, & Lloyd, 2004 Yoder & Layton, 1988
Environmental arrangement strategies—The environment is arranged to promote social communication, initiation, and development (e. g., placing desired materials out of reach and creating a problem-solving situation).	Hwang & Hughes, 2000a, 2000b Matson, Sevin, Fridley, & Love, 1990 Panerai, Ferrante, & Zingale, 2002 Rogers, 1998
Picture schedules and visual supports—The SLP, intervention team, educators, and/or family use pictures to foreshadow activities, allow choices, and depict social communication requests.	MacDuff, Kranz, & McClanahan, 1993 Bryan & Gast, 2000 Watanabe & Sturmey, 2003 Reinhartsen, Garfinkle, & Wolery, 2002 Charlop-Christy, Carpenter, Le, LeBlanc, & Kellert, 2002 Ganz & Simpson, 2004 Johnston, Nelson, Evans, & Palazdo, 2003
Picture exchange communication system (PECS)—A picture or graphic communication system is used to increase functional and spontaneous requests in clients with ASDs.	Bondy & Frost, 1994 Charlop-Christy, Carpenter, Le, LeBlanc, & Kellert, 2002 Ganz & Simpson, 2004

continues

Table 5–4. *continued*

Intervention Perspective	Supportive Evidence
Picture exchange communication system (PECS) *continued*	Johnston, Nelson, Evans, & Palazdo, 2003 Kravits, Kammps, Kemmerer, & Potucek, 2002 Krantz & McClannahan, 1998 Schwartz, Garfinkle, & Bauer, 1998 Ticani, 2004 Yoder & Stone, 2006
Social stories—Printed text is supplemented with picture icons or photographs to provide scripts for appropriate behaviors and social skills.	Charlop-Christy & Kelso, 2003 Krantz & McClannahan, 1998 Sarokoff, Taylor, & Poulson, 2001 Gray, 1995 Barry & Burlew, 2004 Ivey, Heflin, & Alberto, 2004 Kuttler, Miles, & Carson, 1990 Kerr & Durkin, 2004 Parsons & Mitchell, 1999 Wellman et al., 2002
Play and peer mediation—Children with autism spectrum disorders are included in natural play settings with age-matched peers; the adult teaches specific interaction styles to the age-matched peers and also facilitates pragmatic skills in the child with the disorder.	Haring & Lovinger, 1989 Guralnick, 1976 Sainato, Goldstein, & Strain, 1992 Shearer, Kohler, Buchan, & McCullough, 1996 Strain, Kerr, & Ragland, 1979 Odom & Strain, 1984 Oke & Schreibman, 1990 Pierce & Schreibman, 1994 Strain & Kohler, 1998 Taylor, Levin, & Jasper, 1999 Thiemann & Goldstein, 2004
Video modeling—The child with autism spectrum disorder watches a video of a peer or peers engaged in the targeted social skill. The SLP, intervention team, educators, and/or family view and discuss the video multiple times with the child.	Charlop & Milstein, 1989 Charlop-Christy, Le, & Freeman, 2000 Taylor, Levin, & Jasper, 1999
Computerized instruction—The SLP, intervention team, educators, and/or family teach the child with autism spectrum disorder keyboarding skills and computer use for the development of sentence structure, vocal and written responses, vocal imitation, social problem solving, vocabulary, communication initiation, and topic-related communication.	Yamamoto & Miya, 1999 Bernard-Opitz, Sriram, & Sapuan, 1999 Bernard-Opitz, Sriram, & Nakhoda-Sapuan, 2001 Bosseler & Massaro, 2003 Moore & Calvert, 2000, 2003 Hetzroni & Tannous, 2004
Preview learning context and activity—The SLP, intervention team, educators, and/or family spend approximately one hour foreshadowing the day's academic lessons with students with ASD.	Koegel, Koegel, Frea, & Green-Hopkins, 2003

ASD = autism spectrum disorder.

Fluency Remediation

Background

Approximately 2% of adults and 5% of children exhibit fluency disorders. Characteristics of dysfluencies can be part and whole word repetitions, prolongations of sounds, hesitations, muscle tension, and emotional reactions to the dysfluencies. The frequency, duration, type, and severity of dysfluency vary from person to person and from situation to situation. Educational, social, and vocational potential may be affected by dysfluency (Conture & Yaruss, 2007).

General Recommendations

Many speakers report greater benefits from comprehensive approaches than from those that focus only on changes in speech fluency (Yaruss et al., 2002). Approximately 61% of school-aged children who receive services from an SLP show a reduction in the frequency of dysfluency (Conture & Guitar, 1993). Table 5-5 provides the supportive

Table 5–5. Evidence of What Works: Fluency

Intervention Perspective	Supportive Evidence
Cognitive-behavioral treatment regimen designed for relapse management in teens	Blood, 1995
A combination of group and individual treatment for school-age populations; teaches direct strategies for fluent speech (e. g., easy onset, relaxed muscles, prolongations), directly teaches how to modify instances of stuttering when they occur (e. g., pull-outs)	Conture, 1996
Treatment of attitudes, beliefs, and perceptions of teen (i.e., promote cognitive and emotional change)	Daley, Simon, & Burnett-Stolnack, 1995
Interactive videoconferencing with adolescent and adult populations—shape communication behaviors with realistic turn taking and pragmatics	Fosnot, 1993 Sicotte, Lehaux, Fortier-Blanc, & Leblanc, 2003
Multifaceted, individually tailored program for preschool population, focuses on reducing environmental demands, parent-teacher training for affective support and behavior training, and direct teaching of fluency-enhancing strategies	Gottwald & Starkweather, 1995
Parent-conducted program—uses verbal response–contingent stimulation with a school-age population	Lincoln & Onslow (1997)
Parent-conducted program with preschool population	Onslow, Andrews, & Lincoln, 1994
Delayed auditory feedback (but limited generalization) with school-age population	Ryan & Van Kirk Ryan, 1983
Gradual increase in length and complexity of utterances with school-age population	Ryan & Van Kirk Ryan, 1983
Fluency rules program—gives the child "do" statements, rather than "don't" statements, that describe what the child should do to maintain fluency	Runyan & Runyan, 1993
Stuttering modification—changes stuttering characteristics while they occur for school-age populations	Starkweather, Gottwald, & Halfond, 1990
Fluency shaping—teaches skills necessary to speak fluently in school-age populations	Shine, 1994 Meyers & Woodford, 1992

evidence for those clinical approaches that typically are used by school-based SLPs. No single approach is endorsed over another.

Voice Therapy

Background

Ramig and Verdolini (2007) documented that voice disorders affect approximately 10% of the population and are characterized by abnormal pitch, loudness, quality, and resonance. The person with a voice disorder may experience stress, withdrawal, and depression.

General Recommendations

ASHA's (2002b) National Outcomes Measurement System (NOMS) documented that people who receive voice therapy from an SLP makes significant gains on the voice functional communication measures and that more treatment time yields better outcomes. Table 5–6 shows the supportive evidence for those clinical approaches that typically are used by school-based SLPs. No single approach is endorsed over another.

Hearing Loss Treatment

Background

Diefendorf (2007) documented that approximately 11% to 15% of school-aged children exhibit hearing loss. If undetected, hearing loss may have a negative impact on cognitive development, communication competencies, language development, overall child development, literacy, and academic achievement. Early intervention is essential.

General Recommendations

An SLP should be involved with all aspects of communication including oral and sign language development, speech production, voice characteristics, lip reading, and aural habilitation and rehabilitation. Table 5–7, adapted from the work of Carney and Moeller (1998), shows the supportive evidence for those clinical approaches that typically are used by school-based SLPs. No single approach is endorsed over any others.

Augmentative and Alternative Communication Technology

Augmentative, alternative, or assistive devices and services may be used with children who exhibit a variety of communication delays, disorders, or differences. Table 5–8 shows clinical strategies and techniques that have been shown to be effective with all age levels. No one approach is promoted or endorsed over another.

Pediatric Swallowing and Feeding Disorders (Dysphagia)

Background

Arvedson (2006) documented that feeding and swallowing disorders in children may result from congenital or acquired neurological damage, anatomical and structural problems, genetic conditions, systemic illness, and psychosocial and behavioral issues. Approximately 57% of children with cerebral palsy are estimated to have problems with sucking, 38% with swallowing, and 33% with malnutrition.

General Recommendations

Clinical evidence has documented that children with swallowing and feeding problems benefit from services provided by a team of professionals that includes an SLP. Table 5–9 shows the supportive evidence for those clinical approaches that typically are used by swallowing management teams. No single approach is endorsed over any others.

Table 5–6. Evidence of What Works: Voice

Treatment Perspective	Supportive Evidence
Electromyographic biofeedback of laryngeal muscle activity in children	Allen, Bernstein, & Chalt, 1991
Progressive relaxation	Andrews, Warner, & Stewart, 1986
Yawn-sigh	Boone & McFarlane, 1993 Brewer & McCall, 1974
Laryngeal massage	Roy & Leeper, 1993 Roy, Bless, Helsey, & Ford, 1997
Accent method	Fex, Shiromotu, & Hirano, 1994 Kotby, El-Sady, Basiouny, Abou-Rass, & Hegazi, 1991 Smith & Thyme, 1976
Chewing method	Brodnitz & Froeschels, 1954
Vocal intensity reduction	Holbrook, Rolnick, & Bailey, 1974 Lodge & Yanall, 1981
Pitch elevation	Fisher & Logemann, 1970 McFarlane, 1988
Cough reduction	Zwitman & Calcaterra, 1973
Vocal function exercises	Sabol, Lee, & Stempie, 1995 Stempie, Lee, D'Amico, & Picup, 1994
Confidential and resonant voice therapy	Verdolini-Marston, Sandage, & Titze, 1994
Vocal hygiene (education about healthy voice care, optimum use, elimination of abusive habits, increased hydration)	Blood, 1994 Murry & Woodson, 1992 Verdolini-Marston, Burk, Lessac, Glaze, & Caldwell, 1995 Yamaguchi, et al., 1986
Behavioral voice treatment in combination with surgical or other medical management	Koufman & Blalock, 1989 Lancer, Syder, Jones, & LeBoutillier, 1988 Murry & Woodson, 1992 Watterson, Hansen-Magorian, & McFarlane, 1990
Combination of vocal hygiene, abuse reduction, and vocal reeducation	McFarlane & Watterson, 1990 Murry & Woodson, 1992
Vocal abuse reduction program for school-aged children	Johnson, 1995
Vocal hygiene classroom programs for children	Flynn, 1983 Nilson & Schneiderman, 1983
Combined medical, surgical, behavioral, and/or pharmacological approach to increase or decrease vocal fold adduction	Ramig & Verdolini, 1998

Table 5–7. Evidence of What Works: Hearing Impairment Intervention

Intervention Perspective	Supportive Evidence
Sensory and perceptual skill development; wearing aids consistently; increasing auditory perceptual skills; learning to extract electrical cues; learning to extract tactile cues	Strong & Clark, 1992 Hawkins, 1984 Moelier, Donaghy, Besuchaine, Lewis, & Stelmachowicz, 1996 Eilers, Cobo-Lewis, Oiler, & Friedman, 1996 Geers & Brenner, 1994 Miyamoto et al, 1995 Osberger et al., 1991
Language development; enhancing parent-child communication; concept development; comprehension of units of discourse; vocabulary development; expanding world knowledge; developing verbal reasoning skills for literacy development; enhancing self-expression; syntactic, semantic, and pragmatic rules; developing narrative skills	Bodner-Johnson, 1986 Clark, 1994 Davis, Elfenbein, Schum, & Bentler, 1986 Geers & Moog, 1989, 1992 Greenberg, Calderon, & Kusche, 1984 Greenstein, 1975 Luetke-Stahlman & Moeller, 1990, 1996 Moeller et al., 1990 Moeller & McConkey, 1983 Moog & Geers, 1985 Robbins, Osberger, Miyammoto, & Kessler, 1995 Schlesinger & Acree, 1984 Strong & Prinz, 1997
Speech production; increasing vocalization with appropriate timing and vocal tract space characteristics; increasing phonetic and phonemic repertoires; establishing links between perception and production; improving voice and prosody; increasing intelligibility	Eilers & Oiler, 1994 Elfenbein, Hardin-Jones, & Davis, 1994 Fryauf-Bertschy, Tyler, Kelsay, Grantz, & Woodworth, 1997 Higgins, Carney, McCleary, & Rogers, 1996 Osberger, Maso, & Sam, 1993 Tobey, Geers, & Brenner, 1994 Tye-Murray, Spencer, & Woodworth 1995
Academic performance; increase reading and literacy skills; optimize educational achievement with a language base	Schlesinger & Acree, 1984
Social-emotional growth; acceptance of hearing loss; reduce family stress; foster social-emotional development through the school years	Bodner-Johnson, 1986 Greenberg, 1983 Schlesinger & Acree, 1984 Watkins, 1987 White, 1984

Table 5–8. Evidence of What Works: Augmentative and Alternative Communication (AAC) Intervention

Intervention Perspective	Supportive Evidence
Iconic symbols are more easily learned	Wilkinson & McIlvane, 2002
Progression for symbols: real object, color photographs, black-and-white photographs, miniature objects, black- and-white line drawings, Bliss symbols, orthography	Millikin, 1997 Lloyd, Fuller, Loncke, & Bos, 1997
Enhance message timing	Lloyd, Fuller, Loncke, & Bos, 1997
Assist grammatical formulation	Lloyd, Fuller, Loncke, & Bos, 1997
Enhance communication rates	Higginbotham, 1992 Light & Lindsay, 1992 Szeto, Allen, & Littrell, 1993 Venkatagiri, 1993, 1999
Hierarchy of control sites (e.g., fingers and hands before head and feet)	Dowden & Cook, 2002
Direct selection is faster and easier to learn than scanning	Cook & Hussey, 1995 Dowden & Cook, 2002
The role of AAC may vary depending on the course of the disorder	Dowden & Cook, 2002
Decrease in socially inappropriate behaviors and an increase in socially appropriate behaviors with the introduction of AAC	Carr & Durand, 1985 Dropic & Reichle 2001 McEvoy & Neilsen, 2001 Mirenda, 1997a, 1997b Reichle & Wacker, 1993 Robinson & Owens, 1995
Participation model	Beukelman & Mirenda, 1998 Schlosser et al., 2000
Focus on social interaction, making choices and decisions	Light & Gulens, 2000 Krogh & Lindsay, 1999
Cultural sensitivity and recognition of linguistic diversity	Hetzroni & Harris, 1996 Soto, Huer, & Taylor, 1997 Zangari & Kangas, 1997 Parette, VanBiervliet, Reyna, & Heisserer, 1999
Team approach to intervention	Swengel & Marquette, 1997
Feature matching	Glennen, 1997 Quist & Lloyd, 1997
Naturalistic, client- and family-centered approaches	Sigafoos, 1999 Bjorek-Akeson, Granlund, Light, & McNaughton, 2000 Blacksone & Dowden, 2000
Synthesized speech at a rapid rate with fewer pauses	Ratclif, Caughlin, & Lehman, 2002
AAC as a way to facilitate verbal speech	Zangari & Kangas, 1997

Table 5–9. Evidence of What Works: Dysphagia

Intervention Perspective	Supportive Evidence
Use a team approach to assessment that includes an SLP, pediatrician, nutritionist or dietitian, nurse, occupational therapist, physical therapist, psychologist, and social worker	ASHA, 2002 b Drake, O'Donoghue, Bartram, Lindsay, & Greenwood, 1997 Ekberg, 1986 Larnert & Eckberg, 1995 Logemann, 1993a, 1993b, 1998 Ohmae, Logemann, Kaiser, Hanson, & Kahrilas, 1998 Rasley et al., 1993 Robbins & Levine, 1993 Shanahan, Logemann, Rademaker, Pauloski, & Kahrilas, 1993
Evaluate swallowing function parameters including pharyngeal pooling of secretions, premature spillage, laryngeal penetration, aspiration, residue, vocal fold mobility, gag reflex, and laryngeal adductor reflux	Gisel, Birnbaum, & Schwartz, 1998 Willging, 2000
Assess oral pharyngeal and esophageal phases of swallowing using a dynamic instrumental technique including a videoflurosocopic swallow study, endoscopic assessment of swallow function, ultrasonography, and scintigraphy	ASHA, 2002a, 2002b Arvedson & Lefton-Greif, 1998 Balan et al., 1998 Bosma, Hepburn, Josell, & Baker, 1990 Estevao-Costa et al., 2001 Hartnick, Miller, Hartley, & Willging, 2000 Leder & Karas, 2000 Link, Willging, Miller, Cotton, & Rudolph, 2000 Latini et al., 1999 McVeagh, Howman-Giles, & Kemp, 1987 Tolia, Kuhns, & Kauffman, 1993 Weber, Wooldridge, & Baum, 1986 Yang, Loveday, Metrewell, & Sullivan, 1997
Evaluate the lipid-laden macrophage index	Bauer & Lyrene, 1999
Interpretation of videofluoroscopy study that is developmentally appropriate	Newman, Cleveland, Buckman, Hillman, & Jaramillo, 1991
Combine standard endoscopic assessment with a technique that determines laryngeal sensory discrimination thresholds	Link, Willging, Miller, Cotton, & Rudolph, 2000
Test the innervations of the laryngeal adductor reflex by the superior laryngeal nerve	Link, 2000 Liu, Kaplan, Parides, & Close, 2000
Treatment goals should include the following: support adequate nutrition and hydration; minimize risk of pulmonary complications; maximize quality of life; optimize neurodevelopmental potential; develop movements and coordination of the mouth, the respiratory and phonatory system, oral motor function, and support positioning	ASHA, 2002b Logemann, 2000

Table 5–9. *continued*

Intervention Perspective	Supportive Evidence
and seating; develop muscle tone and sensory functions; and promote social-emotional and psychological-behavioral development	
Oral sensorimotor treatment strategies for children with cerebral palsy	Gisel, 1994, 1996 Gisel, Applegate-Ferrante, Benson, & Bosma, 1995, 1996
Range-of-motion exercises for each structure	Veis, Logemann, & Colangelo, 1997 Martin, Logemann, Shaker, & Dodds, 1993
Change timing and level of airway closure	Martin, Logemann, Shaker, & Dodds, 1993 Ohmae, Logemann, Kaiser, Hanson, & Kahrilas, 1996
Change laryngeal motion and cricopharyngeal opening	Kahrilas, Logemann, Drugler, & Glanagan, 1991
Change dietary and feeding patterns	Logemann, 1998 Logemann, 2000
Change swallow physiology through active exercise	Kahrilas et al., 1992 Logemann, 1998 Neuman, 1993
Sensory enhancement	Arvedson & Homer , 2006 Bisch, Logemann, Rademaker, Kahrilas, & Lazarus, 1994 Lazarus, Logemann, & Gibbons, 1993 Lazaras, Lazarus, & Logemann, 1986 Ylvisaker & Logemann, 1998 McPherson et al., 1992
Utensil modifications	Arvedson & Homer, 2006
Caregiver education and training	Arvedson & Homer, 2006
Improve pressure generated by the oral tongue and tongue base during the swallow (effortful swallow)	Pouderoux & Kahrilas, 1995

General Clinical Strategies

Clinical strategies and techniques are available for use by SLPs across a variety of intervention programs regardless of the student's disability type. Table 5–10 presents a summary of such approaches. No one approach is advocated over another.

Table 5–10. Evidence of What Works: General Clinical Strategies

Clinical Strategy	Supportive Evidence
Authentic assessment	Chuney & Burk, 1998 Schraeder, Quinn, Stockman, & Miller, 1999 Stitt & Eger, 2006 ASHA, 2007b
Behavior management—establishing rules, rewards, and consequences; conflict resolution	Orlich, 1980 Canter & Canter, 1985 Curwin & Mendler, 1998 Johnson & Johnson, 1995, 1996 Warner & Bryan, 1995 Kohn, 1996 Cotton, 2005 White, 2004 Webne-Behrman, 2005
Carryover activities or program	Marzano, Pickering, & Pollock, 2001
Clear, specific objectives	Orlich, 1980
Cloze technique—eliciting the target from the client by using an initial carrier phrase followed by a pause (e.g., "The opposite of up is . . .")	Bellon-Harn, Hoffman, & Harn, 2004 Yamashita, 2003
Collaboration	Hedge & Davis, 1995
Cues and prompts (visual, verbal, tactile, prosodic, contextual, and so on)	Chuney & Burk, 1998 Gray, 2005 Hustad & Gearhart, 2004 Klick, 1985 Marzano, Pickering, & Pollock, 2001 Weismer & Hesketh, 1993 Hedge & Maul, 2006a
Cultural competence—respecting the diversity of communication styles among various ethnic groups and cultures	Battle, 1998 ASHA, 2005, 2007b Schraeder, 2001, 2006
Curriculum-based goals	ASHA, 2000 Ehren, 2006 Stitt & Eger, 2006
Data collection—collecting qualitative and quantitative data related to the occurrence of the target behavior	Roth & Worthington, 1996
Developmentally appropriate materials and activities	Chuney & Burk, 1998 Schraeder, 2007
Distributive practice—reviewing past learning	Donovan & Radosevich, 1999
Echo-expansion—echoing what the client said and providing an expanded form (*example:* The child says, "Red truck," and the SLP says, "Red truck—it's a big red truck with yellow wheels")	Scherer & Olswang, 1984 Yoder, Spruytenburg, Edwards, & Davies, 1995
Extended pause time—allowing an extended pause after a question so that the client has time to formulate thoughts into words	Weismer & Schraeder, 1993
Foreshadow—verbalizing the expectation before the action (e.g., "We will use our inside voices and our walking feet")	Hunter, 1985 Canter & Canter, 1985 Barkley, 1987

Table 5–10. *continued*

Clinical Strategy	Supportive Evidence
General and specific corrective feedback	Marzano, Pickering, & Pollock, 2001 Orlich, 1980
General and specific verbal praise	Marzano, Pickering, & Pollock, 2001 Orlich, 1980
Guided practice	Marzano, Pickering, & Pollock, 2001
Guided questions (scaffolding)	Orlich, 1980 Weismer & Schraeder, 1993 Bliss, Askew, & Macrae, 1996 Merritt & Culatta, 1998
Inclusive practices	Villa & Thousand, 1995 Fisher, Shumaker, & Deshler, 2006 Ferguson, 2006 Schraeder, 2007 U.S. Department of Education, 2000
Informal assessment	Miller & Paul, 1995 Swanson, 1996 Poteet, Choate, & Stewart, 1996 Shinn & Hubbard, 1996 Greenwood & Reith, 1996 Wesson & King, 1996 Miller et al., 2005 ASHA, 2007a Schraeder, 2007
Lesson summary with a focus on the objective	Reed, 2005 Tibbets, 1995
Linguistic input at the learner's level	Yoder, Warren, Kim, & Gazdag, 1994 Kuder, 1997
Manage legal paperwork	ASHA, 2002a, 2002b Schraeder, 2007
Massed practice	Donovan & Radosevich, 1999
Model imitation	Garfinkle & Schwartz, 2002 Hedge & Maul, 2006b
Monitor and adjust based on client's needs	Hedge & Maul, 2006
Organize the learning environment	Tessmer & Harris, 1992 Dunlop & Grabinger, 1996 McCoy, 1995a
Proximity praise	Madsen, Becker, & Thomas, 1968 Martin, 1971 Shelton & Meyer, 1977
Reflections on clinical competencies	McCarthy, 2003 ASHA, 2006 Schraeder, 2007
Reinforcement (verbal, tangible, edible)	Marzano, Pickering, & Pollock, 2001
Standardized test use	ASHA, 2007a, 2007b
Technology use	ASHA, 1997 McCoy, 1995

Summary

The call for evidence-based practice began in the medical field in the 1990s and was strengthened in the educational field by mandates in NCLB of 2002. The rigor of peer-reviewed publications was deemed inadequate. A ranking system for levels of evidence was added to the scrutiny of professional literature. The ASHA created a framework for ranking levels of evidence that is specific to the field of communication disorders and sciences. The school-based SLP must consider the mandates of IDEA '04 when applying the concepts of evidence-based practice to clinical work.

Questions for Application and Review

1. What are the three criteria the NRC identified in a framework for evaluating scientific evidence?
2. List the three major characteristics that constitute threats to internal validity.
3. List the four major characteristics that constitute threats to external validity.
4. List two major characteristics that relate to generalization.
5. What is the internationally accepted instrument used by the ASHA for assessing the quality of clinical practice guidelines?
6. What are the two problems that the ASHA Committee on Evidence-Based Practice (ACEBP) identified when reviewing various systems that have been created to evaluate levels of evidence?
7. What are the four levels within the continuum that the ASHA ACEBP created?
8. What makes the continuum created by the ASHA ACEBP unique?
9. What are the two challenges Gillam and Gillam (2006) identified that school-based SLPs face when charged with creating their own evidence base for preferred practice patterns?
10. Under what circumstances would a school need to conduct the type of analysis described by Gillam and Gillam (2006)?

References

The AGREE Collaboration. (2001). *Appraisal of guidelines for research and evaluation (AGREE)*. Retrieved February 3, 2007, from //www.agreecollaboration.org/instrument/

Aldred, C., Green, J., & Adams, C. (2004). A new social communication intervention for children with autism: Pilot randomized controlled treatment study suggesting effectiveness. *Journal of Child Psychology and Psychiatry, and Allied Disciplines, 45,* 1420–1430.

Allen, K. D., Bernstein, B., & Chalt, D. H. (1991). EMG biofeedback treatment of pediatric hyperfunction dysphonia. *Journal of Behavioral Therapy and Experimental Psychiatry, 22*(2), 97–101.

American Speech-Language-Hearing Association. (1997). *Maximizing the provision of appropriate technology services and devices for students in schools* [Technical report]. Available from www.asha.org/policy

American Speech-Language-Hearing Association. (1999). Report: Augmentative and alternative communication. *ASHA, 33*(Suppl. 5), 9–12.

American Speech-Language-Hearing Association. (2000). *Developing educationally relevant IEPs: A technical assistance document for speech-language pathologists.* Rockville, MD: Author.

American Speech-Language-Hearing Association. (2001). Roles of the speech-language pathologist in swallowing and feeding disorders [Technical report]. *ASHA 2002 Desk Reference, 3,* 181–199.

American Speech-Language-Hearing Association. (2002a). *A workload analysis approach to caseload standards in schools.* Rockville, MD: Author.

American Speech-Language-Hearing Association. (2002b). *National outcome measurement system.* Retrieved February 3, 2007, from http://professional.asha.org/resources/NOMS/treatment_outcomes.cfm

American Speech-Language-Hearing Association. (2003). Code of ethics (revised). *ASHA, 23*(Suppl.), 13–15.

American Speech-Language-Hearing Association. (2004a). Auditory integration training. *ASHA, 24*(Suppl.).

American Speech-Language-Hearing Association. (2004b). Examples of evidentiary guidelines for evaluating preponderance of evidence. Retrieved from *ASHA Leader Online,* February 1, 2007, from Mullen, R. (2007, March 6): The state of the evidence: ASHA develops levels of evidence for communication sciences and disorders. *The ASHA Leader, 12*(3), 8–9, 24–25.

American Speech-Language-Hearing Association. (2004c). *Facilitated communication*. Rockville, MD: Author.

American Speech-Language-Hearing Association. (2005). Cultural competence. Retrieved September 6, 2007, from www.asha.org/policy

American Speech-Language-Hearing Association. (2006). *Professional performance review process for the school-based speech-language pathologist*. Retrieved February 1, 2007, from www.asha.org/policy

American Speech-Language-Hearing Association. (2007a). *Directory of speech-language pathology assessment instruments*. Rockville, MD: Author.

American Speech-Language-Hearing Association. (2007b). *Glossary of terms*. Retrieved January 17, 2007, from http://www.asha.org/members/ebp/Glossary.htm

Andrews, S., Warner, J., & Stewart, R. (1986). EMG biofeedback and relaxation in the treatment of hyperfunctional dysphonia. *British Journal of Disorders of Communication, 21*, 353-369.

Arvedson, J. C., & Homer, E. M. (2006). Managing dysphagia in the schools. *The ASHA Leader, 11*(13), 8-9, 28-30.

Arvedson, J. C., & Lefton-Greif, M. (1998). *Pediatric videofluroscopic swallow studies*. San Antonio, TX: Communication Skills Builders.

ASHA Leader. (2007). The state of the evidence: ASHA develops levels of evidence for communication sciences and disorders. *The ASHA Leader, 12*(3), 8-9, 24-25.

Baker, D., Horner, R., Sappington, G., & Ard, W. (2000). A response to Wehmeyer (1999) and a challenge to the field regarding self-determination. *Focus on Autism and Other Developmental Disabilities, 15*, 154.

Balan, K. K., Vinjamuri, S., Maltby, P., Bennett, J., Woods, S., Playfer, J. R., et al. (1998). Gastroesophageal reflux in patients fed by percutaneous endoscopic gastrostomy (PEG): Detection by a simple scintigraphic method. *American Journal of Gastroenterology, 93*, 946-949.

Barkley, S. (1987). *Coaching teachers to higher levels of effectiveness*. Emerson, NJ: Performance Learning Systems.

Barrera, R. D., & Sulzer-Azaroff, B. (1983). An alternating treatment comparison of oral and total communication training programs with echolalic autistic children. *Journal of Applied Behavior Analysis, 16*, 379-394.

Barrera, R. D., Lobatos-Barrera, D., & Sulzer-Azaroff, B. (1980). A simultaneous treatment comparison of three expressive language training programs with a mute autistic child. *Journal of Autism and Developmental Disorders, 10*, 21-37.

Barry, L. M., & Burlew, S. B. (2004). Using social stories to teach choice and play skills to children with autism. *Focus on Autism and Other Developmental Disabilities, 19*, 45-51.

Battle, D. (1998). *Communication disorders in multicultural populations* (2nd ed.). Newton, MA: Butterworth-Heinemann.

Bauer, M. L., & Lyrene, R. K. (1999). Chronic aspiration in children: Evaluation of the lipid-laden macrophage index. *Pediatric Pulmonology, 28*, 79-82.

Bellon-Harn, M. L., Hoffman, P. R., & Harn, W. E. (2004). Use of cloze and contrast word procedures in repeated storybook reading: Targeting multiple domains. *Journal of Communication Disorders, 37*, 53-75.

Bernard-Opitz, V., Sriram, N., & Nakhoda-Sapuan, S. (2001). Enhancing social problem solving in children with autism and normal children through computer-assisted instruction. *Journal of Autism and Developmental Disorders, 31*, 377-384.

Bernard-Opitz, V., Sriram, N., & Sapaun, S. (1999). Enhancing vocal imitation in children with autism using the IBM Speechviewer. *Autism, 3*, 131-147.

Bernthal, J., & Bankson, N. (2004). *Articulation and phonological disorders* (5th ed.). Boston: Allyn & Bacon.

Beukelman, D., & Mirenda, P. (1998). Principles of assessment. In D. Beukelman & P. Mirenda (Eds.), *Augmentative and alternative communication* (2nd ed., pp. 145-169). Baltimore: Brookes.

Bisch, E. M., Logemann, J. A., Rademaker, A. W., Kahrilas, P. J., & Lazarus, C. L. (1994). Pharyngeal effects of bolus volume, viscosity and temperature in patients with dysphagia resulting from neurologic impairment and in normal subjects. *Journal of Speech and Hearing Research, 3*, 1041-1049.

Bjorek-Akeson, E., Granlund, E., Light, J., & McNaughton, D. (2000). Goal setting and problem solving with AAC users and families. In *Proceedings of the 9th Biennial Conference of the International Society for AAC* (pp. 50-52). Washington, DC: ISAAC.

Blackstone, S., & Dowden, P. (2000). Two to tango: AAC users and their communication partners. In *Proceedings of the 9th Biennial Conference of the International Society for AAC* (pp. 129-131). Washington, DC: ISAAC.

Bliss, J., Askew, M., & Macrae, S. (1996). Effective teaching and learning: Scaffolding revisited. *Oxford Review of Education, 22*(1), 37-67.

Blood, G. W. (1994). Efficacy of a computer-assisted voice treatment protocol. *American Journal of Speech-Language Pathology, 3*(1), 57-66.

Blood, G. (1995). POWER: Relapse management with adolescents who stutter. *Language, Speech, and Hearing Services in Schools, 26,* 169-179.

Blosser, J. (2006). *Partnering with teachers for speech-language service delivery.* Retrieved March 23, 2006, from http://www.speechpathology.com

Bodner-Johnson, B. (1986). The family environment and achievement of deaf students: A discriminate analysis. *Exceptional Children, 53,* 443-449.

Bondy, A., & Frost, L. (1994). The Picture Exchange Communication System. *Focus on Autistic Behavior, 9,* 1-9.

Boone, D., & McFarlane, S. (1993). A critical view of the yawn-sigh as a voice therapy technique. *Journal of Voice, 7,* 75-80.

Bopp, K. D., Brown, K. E., & Mirenda, P. (2004). Speech-language pathologists' roles in the delivery of positive behavior support for individuals with developmental disabilities. *American Journal of Speech-Language Pathology, 13,* 5-19.

Bosma, J. F., Hepburn, L. G., Josell, S. D., & Baker, K. (1990). Ultrasound demonstration of tongue motions during suckle feeding. *Developmental Medicine and Child Neurology, 32,* 223-229.

Bosseler, A., & Massaro, D. W. (2003). Development and evaluation of a computer-animated tutor for vocabulary and language learning in children with autism. *Journal of Autism and Developmental Disorders, 33,* 653-672.

Brady, N. (2000). Improved comprehension of object names following voice output communication aid use: Two case studies. *Augmentative and Alternative Communication, 16,* 197-204.

Brewer, D. W., & McCall, G. N. (1974). Visible laryngeal changes during voice therapy. *Annals of Otology, Rhinology, and Laryngology, 83,* 423-427.

Brodnitz, F. S., & Froeschels, E. (1954). Treatment of nodules of vocal cords by chewing method. *Archives of Otolaryngology, 59*(5), 560-565.

Bryan, L. C., & Gast, D. L. (2000). Teaching on-task and on-schedule behaviors to higher functioning children with autism via picture activity schedules. *Journal of Autism and Developmental Disorders, 30,* 553-567.

Camarata, S. (1993). The application of naturalistic conversation training to speech production in children with specific disabilities. *Journal of Applied Behavioral Analysis, 26,* 173-182.

Canter, L., & Canter, M. (1985). *Assertive discipline.* Santa Monica, CA: Canter Associates.

Carney, A. E., & Moeller, M. P. (1998). Treatment efficacy: Hearing loss in children. *Journal of Speech, Language, and Hearing Research, 41,* S61-S84.

Caro, P., & Snell, M. (1989). Characteristics of teaching communication to people with moderate and severe disabilities. *Education and Training in Mental Retardation, 24,* 63-77.

Carr, E. G., Dunlap, G., Horner, R. H., Koegel, R. L., Turnbull, A. P., Sailor, W., et al. (2002). Positive behavior support: Evolution of an applied science. *Journal of Positive Behavior Interventions, 4*(1), 4-16, 20.

Carr, E., & Durand, M. (1985). Reducing behavior problems through functional communication training. *Journal of Applied Behavior Analysis, 18,* 111-126.

Charlop, M. H., & Milstein, J. P. (1989). Teaching autistic children conversational speech using video modeling. *Journal of Applied Behavior Analysis, 22,* 275-285.

Charlop, M. H., Schreibman, L., & Thibodeau, M. G. (1985). Increasing spontaneous verbal responding in autistic children using a time delay procedure. *Journal of Applied Behavior Analysis, 18,* 155-166.

Charlop-Christy, M. H., Carpenter, M., Le, L., LeBlanc, L. A., & Kellert, K. (2002). Using the Picture Exchange Communication System with children with autism: Assessment of PECS acquisition, speech, social-communicative behavior, and problem behavior. *Journal of Applied Behavior Analysis, 35,* 213-231.

Charlop-Christy, M. H., & Kelso, S. E. (2003). Teaching children with autism conversational speech using a cue card/written script program. *Education and Treatment of Children, 26,* 103-127.

Charlop-Christy, M. H., Le, L., & Freeman, K. A. (2000). A comparison of video modeling with in vivo modeling for teaching children with autism. *Journal of Autism and Developmental Disorders, 30,* 537-552.

Chuney, A. L., & Burk, T. L. (1998). *Teaching oral communication in grades K-8.* Boston: Allyn & Bacon.

Clark, T. (1994). SKI*HI: Applications for home-based intervention. In J. Rousch & N. Matkin (Eds.), *Infants and toddlers with hearing loss: Family-centered assessment and intervention* (pp. 237-251). Baltimore: York Press.

Cohen, W., Hodson, A., O'Hare, A., Boyle, J., Durrani, T., McCartney, E., et al. (2005). Effects of computer-based intervention through acoustically modified speech (Fast ForWord) in severe mixed receptive-expressive language impairment: Outcomes from a randomized controlled trial. *Journal of Speech, Language, and Hearing Research, 48*(3), 715-729.

Conture, E. G. (1996). Treatment efficacy: Stuttering. *Journal of Speech and Hearing Research, 39,* S18-S26.

Conture, E., & Guitar, B. (1993). Evaluating efficacy of treatment of stuttering: School-age children. *Journal of Fluency Disorders, 18,* 253-287.

Conture, E. G., & Yaruss, J. S. (2007). *Treatment efficacy summary: Stuttering*. Rockville, MD: American Speech-Language-Hearing Association.

Cook, A., & Hussey, S. (1995). *Assistive technologies: Principles and practice*. St. Louis: Mosby.

Cotton, K. (2005). *School wide and classroom discipline*. Retrieved April 1, 2007, from http://www.nwrel.org/scpd/sirs/5/co9.html

Curwin, R., & Mendler, A. (1988). *Discipline with dignity*. Alexandria, VA: Association for Supervision and Curriculum Development.

Daly, D., Simon, C., & Burnett-Stolnack, M. (1995). Helping adolescents who stutter to focus on fluency. *Language, Speech, and Hearing Services in Schools, 26*, 162–168.

Davis, J. M., Elfenbein, J. L. Schum, R., & Bentler, R. (1986). Effects of mild and moderate hearing impairments on language, educational, and psychosocial behavior of children. *Journal of Speech and Hearing Disorders, 51*, 53–62.

Diefendorf, A. (2007). *Treatment efficacy summary: Hearing loss in children*. Rockville, MD: American Speech-Language-Hearing Association.

Donovan, J., & Radosevich, D. (1999). A meta-analytic review of distribution of practice effect: Now you see it, now you don't. *Journal of Applied Psychology, 84*(5), 795–805.

Dowden, P., & Cook, A. (2002). Choosing effective selection techniques for beginning communicators. In J. Reichle, D. Beukelman, & J. Light (Eds.), *Exemplary practices for beginning communicators: Implications for AAC* (pp. 395–431). Baltimore: Brookes.

Drake, W., O'Donoghue, S., Bartram, C., Lindsay, J., & Greenwood, R. (1997). Eating in side-lying facilitates rehabilitation in neurogenic dysphagia. *Brain Injury, 11*, 137–142.

Dropic, P., & Reichle, J. (2001). Developing an intervention strategy to replace challenging behavior used to escape undesired activities: A case study. *Newsletter of the ASHA Special Interest Division 12: Augmentative and Alternative Communication, 10*(1), 6–8.

Dunlap, J. C., & Grabinger, R. S. (1996). Rich environments for active learning in the higher education classroom. In B. G. Wilson (Ed.), *Constructivist learning environments: Case studies in instructional design* (pp. 65–82). Englewood Cliffs, NJ: Educational Technology Publications.

Durand, V. M., & Carr, E. G., (1991). Functional communication training to reduce challenging behavior: Maintenance and application in new settings. *Journal of Applied Behavior Analysis, 24*, 251–264.

Durand, V. M., & Carr, E. G. (1992). An analysis of maintenance following functional communication training. *Journal of Applied Behavior Analysis, 25*, 777–794.

Ehren, B. J. (2006). *Curriculum-relevant therapy with adolescents*. Retrieved April 1, 2007, from: http://www.speechpathology.com

Eilers, R. E., & Oiler, D. K. (1994). Infant vocalizations and the early diagnosis of severe hearing impairment. *Journal of Pediatrics, 124*, 199–203.

Eliers, R. E., Cobo-Lewis, A. B., Oiler, D. K., & Friedman, K. E. (1996). A longitudinal evaluation of the speech perception capabilities of children using multichannel tactile vo-coders. *Journal of Speech and Hearing Research, 39*, 518–533.

Ekberg, O. (1986). Posture of the head and pharyngeal swallowing. *Acta Radiologica Diagnosis, 27*, 691–696.

Elfenbein, J. L., Hardin-Jones, M. A., & Davis, J. M. (1994). Oral communication skills of children who are hard of hearing. *Journal of Speech and Hearing Research, 37*, 216–226.

Ellis Weismer, S., & Murray-Branch, J. (1989). Modeling versus modeling plus evoked production training: A comparison of two language intervention methods. *Journal of Speech, Language, and Hearing Research, 40*, 5–19.

Estevao-Costa, J., Campos, M., Dias, J. A., Trindade, E., Medina, A. M., & Carval, J. L. (2001). Delayed gastric emptying and gastroesophageal reflux: A pathophysiologic relationship. *Journal of Pediatric Gastroenterology and Nutrition, 32*, 471–474.

Ewing, S. (1999). Group process, group dynamics, and group techniques with neurogenic communication disorders. In R. Elman (Ed.), *Group treatment of neurogenic communication disorders* (pp. 9–17). Boston: Butterworth-Heineman.

Ferguson, M. L. (2006). *Designing intervention for academically diverse classrooms: Differentiated instruction techniques for speech-language pathologists*. Retrieved April 26, 2006, from http://www.speechpathology.com

Fex, F., Fex, S., Shiromoto, O., & Hirano, M. (1994). Acoustic analysis of functional dysphonia: Before and after voice therapy (accent method). *Journal of Voice, 8*, 163–167.

Fey, M. (1986). *Language intervention with young children*. San Diego, CA: College-Hill Press.

Fey, M., Cleave, P., & Long, S. (1997). Facilitation in children with language impairments: Phase 2. *Journal of Speech, Language, and Hearing Research, 40*, 5–19.

Fisher, H. B., & Logemann, J. A. (1970). Objective evaluation of therapy for vocal nodules: A case report.

Journal of Speech and Hearing Disorders, 35, 277–285.

Fisher, J. B., Shumaker, J. B., & Deshler, D. D. (1996). *Searching for validated inclusive practices: A review of the literature* (pp. 123–155). In E. Meyen, G. Vergason, & R. Whelan (Eds.), *Strategies for teaching exceptional children in inclusive settings.* Denver, CO: Love.

Flynn, P. T. (1983). Speech-language pathologists and primary prevention: From idea to action. *Language, Speech, and Hearing Services in Schools, 14,* 99–104.

Fosnot, S. (1993). Research design for examining treatment efficacy in fluency disorders. *Journal of Fluency Disorders, 18,* 221–251.

Frea, W. D., Arnold, C., & Vittimberga, G. I. (2001). A demonstration of the effects of augmentative communication on the extreme aggressive behavior of a child with autism within an integrated preschool setting. *Journal of Positive Behavior Interventions, 3,* 194–198.

Fryauf-Bertschy, H., Tyler, R. S., Kelsay, D. M., Grantz, B. J., & Woodworth, G. G. (1997). Cochlear implant use by prelingually deafened children: The influences of age at implant and length of device use. *Journal of Speech and Hearing Research, 40,* 183–199.

Ganz, J. B., & Simpson, R. L. (2004). Effects on communicative requesting and speech development of the Picture Exchange Communication System in children with characteristics of autism. *Journal of Autism and Developmental Disorders, 34,* 395–409.

Garfinkle, A., & Schwartz, S. (2002). Peer imitation: Increasing social interactions in children with autism and other developmental disabilities in inclusive preschool classrooms. *Topics in Early Childhood Special Education, 23*(2), 77–89.

Garrison-Harrell, L., Kamps, D., & Kravits, T. (1997). The effects of peer networks on social-communicative behaviors for students with autism. *Focus on Autism and Other Developmental Disabilities, 12,* 241–254.

Geers, A. E., & Moog, J. S. (1989). Factors predictive of the development of literacy in profoundly hearing-impaired adolescents. *Volta Review, 91,* 69–86.

Geers, A. E., & Brenner, C. (1994). Speech perception results: Audition and lip-reading enhancement. *Volta Review, 96,* 97–108.

Geers, A. E., & Moog, J. S. (1992). Speech perception and production skills of students with impaired hearing from oral and total communication education settings. *Journal of Speech and Hearing Research, 35,* 1384–1393.

Geirut, J. (1998). Treatment efficacy: Functional phonological disorders in children. *Journal of Speech, Language, and Hearing Research, 41,* 85–100.

Gersten, R., & Brengelman, S. (1996). The quest to translate research into classroom practice. *Remedial and Special Education, 17,* 67–74.

Gierut, J. (2007). *Treatment efficacy summary: Phonological disorders in children.* Rockville, MD: American Speech-Language-Hearing Association.

Gierut, J. (2001). Complexity in phonological treatment: Clinical factors. *Language, Speech, and Hearing Services in Schools, 32,* 229–241.

Gierut, J. A. (2005). Phonological intervention: The how or the what? In A. Kamhi & K. Pollock (Eds.), *Phonological disorders in children: Clinical decision making in assessment and intervention* (pp. 201–210). Baltimore: Brookes.

Gillam, R., Loeb, D., Friel-Patti, S., Hoffman, L., Brandel, J., Champlin, C., et al. (2005, November). *Comparing language intervention outcomes.* Seminar presented at annual convention of the American Speech-Language-Hearing Association, San Diego, CA.

Gillam, S. L., & Gillam, R. B., (2006). Making evidence-based decisions about child language intervention in schools. *Language, Speech, and Hearing Services in Schools, 37,* 304–315.

Gillon, G. T. (2005). Facilitating phoneme awareness development in 3–4-year-old children with speech impairment. *Language, Speech, and Hearing Services in Schools, 36,* 308–324.

Gisel, E. (1994). Oral-motor skills following sensorimotor intervention in the moderately eating-impaired child with cerebral palsy. *Dysphagia, 9*(3), 180–192.

Gisel, E. G. (1996). Effect of oral sensorimotor treatment on measures of growth and efficiency of eating in the moderately eating-impaired child with cerebral palsy. *Dysphagia, 11*(1), 48–58.

Gisel, E. G., Applegate-Ferrante, T., Benson, J., & Bosma, J. (1995). Effect of oral sensorimotor treatment on measures of growth, eating, efficiency and aspiration in the dysphagic child with cerebral palsy. *Developmental Medicine and Child Neurology, 37,* 528–543.

Gisel, E., Applegate-Ferrante, T., Benson, J., & Bosma, J. (1996). Oral-motor skills following sensorimotor therapy in two groups of moderately dysphagic children with cerebral palsy: Aspiration vs. nonaspiration. *Dysphagia, 11,* 59–71.

Gisel, E. G., Birnbaum, R., & Schwartz, S. (1998). Feeding impairments in children: Diagnosis and effective intervention. *International Journal of Orofacial Myology, 24,* 27–33.

Glennen, S. (1997). Augmentative and alternative communication assessment strategies. In S. Glennen & D. Decoste (Eds.), *Handbook of augmentative and alternative communication* (pp. 140-192). San Diego, CA: Singular.

Goldstein, H., & Prelock, P. (2007). *Treatment efficacy summary: Child language disorders*. Rockville, MD: American Speech-Language-Hearing Association.

Gorman, C. (2007, Feb. 26). Are doctors just playing hunches? *Time, 169*(9), 52-54.

Gottwald, S., & Starkweather, C. (1995). Fluency intervention for preschoolers and their families in the public schools. *Language, Speech, and Hearing Services in Schools, 26*, 117-126.

Gray, C. A. (1995). Teaching children with autism to "read" social situations. In K. Quill (Ed.), *Teaching children with autism: Strategies to enhance communications and socialization* (pp. 219-241). Albany, NY: Delmar.

Gray, S. (2005). Word learning by preschoolers with specific language impairment. *Journal of Speech, Language, and Hearing, 48*, 1452-1467.

Greenberg, M. (1983). Family stress and child competence: The effects of early intervention for families with deaf infants. *American Annals of the Deaf, 128*, 407-417.

Greenberg, M. T., Calderon, R., & Kusche, C. (1984). Early intervention using simultaneous communication with deaf infants: The effects on communication with deaf infants: The effects on communicative development. *Child Development, 55*, 607-616.

Greenspan, S. I., & Wieder, S. (1997). Developmental patterns and outcomes in infants and children with disorders in relating and communicating: A chart review of 200 cases of children with autistic spectrum diagnoses. *Journal of Developmental and Learning Disorders, 1*, 87-141.

Greenstein, J. (1975). *Methods of fostering language development in deaf infants: Final report* (BBB00581). Washington, DC: Bureau of Education for the Handicapped (DHEW/OE).

Greenwood, C. R., & Reith, H. J. (1996). *Current dimensions of technology-based assessment in special education* (pp. 279-292). In E. Meyen, G. Vergason, & R. Whelan (Eds.), *Strategies for teaching exceptional children in inclusive settings*. Denver, CO: Love.

Guralnick, J. J. (1976). The value of integrating handicapped and nonhandicapped preschool children. *American Journal of Orthopsychiatry, 46*, 236-245.

Haring, T., & Lovinger, L. (1989). Promoting social interaction through teaching generalized play initiation responses to preschool children with autism.

Journal of the Association for Persons with Severe Handicaps, 14(1), 58-67.

Hart, B. (1985). Naturalistic language training strategies. In S. Warren & A. Rogers-Warren (Eds.), *Teaching functional language* (pp. 63-88). Baltimore: University Park Press.

Hart, B., & Risley, T. (1975). In vivo language intervention: Unanticipated general effects. *Journal of Applied Behavioral Analysis, 13*, 411-420.

Hartnick, C., Miller, C., Hartley, B., & Willging, J. (2000). Pediatric fiberoptic endoscopic evaluation of swallowing. *Annals of Otorhinology and Laryngology, 109*, 996-999.

Hawkins, D. (1984). Comparisons of speech recognition in noise by mildly-to-moderately hearing-impaired children using hearing aids and FM systems. *Journal of Speech and Hearing Disorders, 49*, 409-418.

Hedge, M. N., & Davis, D. (1995). *Clinical methods and practicum in speech-language pathology*. San Diego, CA: Singular.

Hedge, M. N., & Maul, C. A. (2006). *Language disorders in children: An evidence-based approach to assessment and treatment*. Boston: Pearson Education.

Hemmeter, M., Ault, M. Collins, B., & Meyer, S. (1996). The effects of teaching-implemented language instruction within free time activities. *Education and Training in Mental Retardation and Developmental Disabilities, 31*, 203-212.

Hetzroni, O., & Harris, O. (1996). Cultural aspects in the development of AAC users. *Augmentative and Alternative Communication, 12*, 52-58.

Hetzroni, O. E., & Tannous, J. (2004). Effects of a computer based intervention program on the communicative functions of children with autism. *Journal of Autism and Developmental Disorders, 34*, 95-113.

Higginbotham, J. (1992). Evaluation of keystroke savings across five assistive communication technologies. *Augmentative and Alternative Communication, 8*, 258-272.

Higgins, M. B., Carney, A. E., McCleary, E., & Rogers, S. (1996). Negative intraoral air pressures of deaf children with cochlear implants: Physiology, phonology, and treatment. *Journal of Speech and Hearing Research, 39*, 957-967.

Hodson, B., & Paden, E. (1991). *Targeting intelligible speech: A phonological approach to remediation* (2nd ed.). Austin, TX: Pro-Ed.

Holbrook, A., Rolnick, M., & Baily, C. W. (1974). Treatment of vocal abuse disorders using a vocal intensity controller. *Journal of Speech and Hearing Disorders, 39*, 298-303.

Holland, A. (1995, April). *Current realities of aphasia rehabilitation: Time constraints, documentation demands and functional outcomes.* Paper presented at an Inservice Training at the Mid-America Rehabilitation Hospital, Overland Park, KS.

Holland, A. I., Fromm, D. S., DeRuyter, F., & Stein, M. (1996). Treatment efficacy: Aphasia. *Journal of Speech and Hearing Research, 39,* 27–39.

Hook, P. E., Macaruso, P., & Jones, S. (2001). Efficacy of FastForWord training on facilitating acquisition of reading skills by children with reading difficulties: A longitudinal study. *Annals of Dyslexia, 51,* 75–96.

Horner, R., Albin, R., Sprague, J., & Todd, A. (2000). Positive behavior support for students with severe disabilities. In M. Snell & F. Brown (Eds.), *Instruction of students with severe disabilities* (5th ed., pp. 207–243). Upper Saddle River, NJ: Prentice-Hall.

Horner, R. H., Day, H. M., Sprague, J. R., O'Brien, M., & Heathfield, L. T. (1991). Interspersed requests: A non-aversive procedure for reducing aggression and self injury during instruction. *Journal of Applied Behavior Analysis, 24,* 265–268.

Howell, J., & Dean, E. (1994). *Treating phonological disorders in children. Metaphon: Theory to practice* (2nd ed.). London: Whurr.

Hunter, M. (1985). *Mastery teaching.* El Segundo, CA: TIP Publications.

Hustad, K., & Gearhart, K. (2004). Listener attitudes toward individuals with cerebral palsy who use speech supplemental strategies. *American Journal of Speech-Language Pathology, 13,* 168–181.

Hwang, B., & Hughes, C. (2000a). The effects of social interactive training on early social communicative skills of children with autism. *Journal of Autism and Developmental Disorders, 30,* 331–343.

Hwang, B., & Hughes, C. (2000b). Increasing early social-communicative skills of preverbal preschool children with autism through social interactive training. *Journal of the Association for Persons with Severe Handicaps, 25,* 18–28.

Ivey, M. L., Heflin, J., & Alberto, P. (2004). The use of social stories to promote independent behaviors in novel events for children with PDD-NOS. *Focus on Autism and Other Developmental Disabilities, 19,* 164–176.

Jacoby, G. P., Lee, L., Kummer, A., W., Levin, L., & Creaghead, N.A. (2002). The number of individual treatment units necessary to facilitate functional communication improvements in the speech and language of young children. *American Journal of Speech-Language Pathology, 11,* 370–380.

Johnson, D. W. & Johnson, R. T. (1995). *Reducing school violence through conflict resolution.* Alexandria, VA: Association for Supervision and Curriculum Development.

Johnson, D. W., & Johnson, R. T. (1996). Peacemakers: Teaching students to resolve their own and schoolmates' conflicts. In E. Meyen, G. Vergason, & R. Whelan (Eds.), *Strategies for teaching exceptional children in inclusive settings* (pp. 311–328). Denver, CO: Love.

Johnston, S., Nelson, C., Evans, J., & Palazolo, K. (2003). The use of visual supports in teaching young children with autism spectrum disorder to initiate interactions. *Augmentative and Alternative Communication, 19,* 86–103.

Johnson, T. S. (1995). Vocal abuse reduction program. New York: Taylor & Francis.

Justice, L. M., & Fey, M. E. (2004, September 21). Evidence-based practice in schools: Integrating craft and theory with science and data. *The ASHA Leader,* pp. 4–5, 30–32.

Kahrilas, P. J., Logemann, J. A., Krugler, C., & Glanagan, E. (1991). Volitional augmentation of upper esophageal sphincter opening during swallowing. *American Journal of Physiology, 260,* G450–G456.

Kaiser, A. (1993). Functional language. In M. Snel (Ed.), *Instruction of students with severe disabilities* (pp. 347–379). New York: Macmillan.

Kaiser, A. P., Yoder, P., & Keetz, A. (1992). Evaluating milieu teaching. In S. F. Warren & J. Reichle (Eds.), *Causes and effects in communication and language intervention* (pp. 9–47). Baltimore: Brookes.

Kamhi, A. (1994). Toward a theory of clinical expertise in speech-language pathology. *Language, Speech, and Hearing Services in Schools, 25,* 115–119.

Kamhi, A. (1999). To use or not to use: Factors that influence the selection of new treatment approaches. *Language, Speech, and Hearing Services in Schools, 30,* 92–98.

Kamhi, A. G. (2006). Treatment decisions for children with speech-sound disorders. *Language, Speech, and Hearing Services in Schools, 37(4),* 271–279.

Kerr, S., & Durkin, K. (2004). Understanding of thought bubbles as mental representations in children with autism: Implications for theory of mind. *Journal of Autism and Developmental Disorders, 34,* 637–648.

Kim, Y., Yang, Y., & Hwang, B. (2001). Generalization effects of script-based intervention on language expression of preschool children with language disorders. *Education and Training in Mental Retardation and Developmental Disabilities, 36,* 411–423.

Klick, S. (1985). Adapted cuing technique for use in treatment of dyspraxia. *Language, Speech, and Hearing Services in Schools, 16,* 256-259.

Koegel, L. K. (1995). Communication and language intervention. In R. Koegel & L. Koegel (Eds.), *Teaching children with autism* (pp. 17-32). Baltimore: Brookes.

Koegel, R. L., Camarata, S., Koegel, L., Ben-Tall, A., & Smith, A. (1998). Increasing speech intelligibility in children with autism. *Journal of Autism and Developmental Disorders, 28,* 241-251.

Koegel, L. K., Koegel, R. L., Frea, W., & Green-Hopkins, I. (2003). Priming as a method of coordinating educational services for students with autism. *Language, Speech, and Hearing Services in Schools, 34,* 228-235.

Koegel, R. L., O'Dell, M. C., & Koegel, L. K. (1987). A natural language paradigm for teaching nonverbal autistic children. *Journal of Autism and Developmental Disorders, 17,* 187-199.

Kohn, A. (1996). *Beyond discipline from compliance to community.* Alexandria, VA: Association for Supervision and Curriculum Development.

Kotby, M., El-Sady, S., Basiouny, S., Abou-Rass, Y., & Hegazi, M. (1991). Efficacy of the accent method of voice therapy. *Journal of Voice, 5,* 316-320.

Koufman, J., & Blalock, P. D. (1989). Is voice rest never indicated? *Journal of Voice, 3,* 87-91.

Kouri, T. (2005). Lexical training through modeling and elicitation procedures with late talkers who have specific language impairment and developmental delays. *Journal of Speech, Language, and Hearing Research, 48,* 157-172.

Krantz, P. J., & McClannahan, L. E. (1998). Social interaction skills for children with autism: A script fading procedure for beginning readers. *Journal of Applied Behavior Analysis, 31,* 191-202.

Kravits, T. R., Kammps, D. M., Kemmerer, K., & Potucek, J. (2002). Brief report: Increasing the communication skills for an elementary-aged student with autism using the Picture Exchange Communication System. *Journal of Autism and Developmental Disorders, 32,* 225-230.

Krogh, K., & Lindsay, P. (1999). Including people with disabilities in research: Implications for the field of augmentative and alternative communication. *Augmentative and Alternative Communication, 15,* 222-223.

Kuder, S. J. (1997). *Teaching students with language and communication disabilities.* Boston: Allyn & Bacon.

Kuttler, S., Miles, B. S., & Carson, J. K. (1999). The use of social stories to reduce precursors to tantrum behavior in a student with autism. *Focus on Autism and Other Developmental Disabilities, 13,* 176-182.

Lalli, J. S., Casey, S., & Kates, K. (1995). Reducing escape behavior and increasing task completion with functional communication training, extinction, and response chaining. *Journal of Applied Behavior Analysis, 28,* 261-268.

Lancer, J. M., Syder, D., Jones, A. S., & LeBoutillier, A. (1988). The outcomes of different management patterns of vocal cord nodules. *Journal of Laryngology and Otology, 102,* 423-427.

Larnert, G., & Ekberg, O. (1995). Positioning improves the oral and pharyngeal swallowing function in children with cerebral palsy. *Acta Padiatrica, 84,* 689-692.

Latini, G., Del Vecchio, A., De Mitri, B., Glannuzzi, R., Presta, G., Quartulli, H., et al. (1999). Scintigraphic evaluation of gastroesophageal reflux in newborns. *La Pediatria Medica e Chirurgica, 21,* 115-117.

Law, J., Garrett, Z., & Nye, C. (2004). Speech and language therapy interventions for children with primary speech and language delay or disorder. *Cochrane Database of Systematic Reviews, 3,* CD004110. Retrieved February 3, 2007, from http://www.cochrane.org/review/clibacress.htm

Layton, T. (1988). Language training with autistic children using four different modes of presentation. *Journal of Communication Disorders, 21,* 333-350.

Lazarus, C., Logemann, J. A., & Gibbons, P. (1993). Effects of maneuvers on swallowing function in a dysphagic oral cancer patient. *Head & Neck, 15,* 419-424.

Lazsaras, G., Lazarus, C., & Logemann, J. A. (1986). Impact of thermal stimulation on the triggering of the swallowing reflex. *Dysphagia, 1,* 73-77.

Lazarus, C. L., Logemann, J. A., Rademaker, A. W., Kahrilas, P. J., Pajak, T., Lazar, R., et al. (1993). Effects of bolus volume, viscosity and repeated swallows in nonstroke subjects and stroke patients. *Archives of Physical Medicine and Rehabilitation, 74,* 1066-1070.

Leder, S. B., & Karas, D. E. (2000). Fiberoptic endoscopic evaluation of swallowing in the pediatric population. *Laryngoscope, 110*(7), 1132-1136.

Lewy, A. L., & Dawson, G. (1992). Social stimulation and joint attention in young autistic children. *Journal of Abnormal Child Psychology, 20,* 555-566.

Light, J., & Gulens, M. (2000). Rebuilding communicative competence and self-determination. In D. Beukelman, K. Yourston, & J. Reichle (Eds.), *Augmentative and alternative communications for adults with acquired neurologic disorders* (pp. 137-179). Baltimore: Brookes.

Light, J., & Lindsay, P. (1992). Message-encoding techniques for augmentative communication systems: The recall performance of adults with severe speech impairments. *Journal of Speech and Hearing Research, 35,* 853-864.

Light, J., Roberts, B., DiMarco, R., & Greiner, N. (1998). Augmentative and alternative communication to support receptive and expressive language for people with autism. *Journal of Communication Disorders, 31,* 153-180.

Lincoln, M., & Onslow, M. (1997. Long-term outcome of early intervention for stuttering. *American Journal of Speech-Language Pathology, 6*(1), 51-58.

Link, D. T., Willging, J., Miller, C. K., Cotton, R., & Rudolph, C. D. (2000). Pediatric laryngopharyngeal sensory during flexible endoscopic evaluation of swallowing: Feasible and correlative. *Annals of Otology, Rhinology, and Laryngology, 109,* 899-905.

Liu, H., Kaplan, S., Parides, M., & Close, L. (2000). Laryngopharyngeal sensory deficits in patients with laryngopharyngeal reflux and dysphagia. *Annals of Otorhinology and Laryngology, 109,* 1000-1006.

Lloyd, L., Fuller, D., Loncke, F., & Bos, H. (1997). Introduction to AAC symbols. In L. Lloyd, D. Fuller, & H. Arvidson (Eds.), *Augmentative and Alternative Communication* (pp. 43-47). Boston: Allyn & Bacon.

Lodge, J., & Yarnall, G. (1981). A case study of vocal volume reduction. *Journal of Speech and Hearing Disorders, 46,* 317-320.

Lof, G., & Watson, M. (2005, November). *Survey of universities teaching oral motor exercises and other procedures.* Poster session at the annual convention of the American Speech-Language-Hearing Association, San Diego, CA.

Logemann, J. A. (1993a). The dysphagia diagnostic procedure as a treatment efficacy trial. *Clinics in Communication Disorders, 3,* 1-10.

Logemann, J. A. (1993b). *A manual for videofluoroscopic evaluation of swallowing* (2nd ed.). Austin, TX: Pro-Ed.

Logemann, J. A. (1998). *Evaluation and treatment of swallowing disorders* (2nd ed.). Austin, TX: Pro-Ed.

Logemann, J. A. (2000). Therapy for children with swallowing disorders in educational settings. *Language, Speech, and Hearing Services in the Schools, 31,* 50-55.

Luetke-Stahlman, B., & Moeller, M. P. (1990). Enhancing parents' use of SEE-2: Progress and retention. *American Annals of the Deaf, 135,* 371-378.

MacDuff, G. S., Krantz, P. J., & McClanahan, L. E. (1993). Teaching children with autism to use photographic activity schedules: Maintenance and generalization of complex response chains. *Journal of Applied Behavior Analysis, 26,* 89-97.

Madsen, C. H., Becker, W. C., & Thomas, D. R. (1968). Rules praise, and ignoring: Elements of elementary classroom control. *Journal of Applied Behavior Analysis, 1*(2), 139-150.

Mahoney, G., & Perales, F. (2005). Relationship-focus early intervention with children with pervasive developmental disorders and other disabilities: A comparative study. *Journal of Developmental and Behavioral Pediatrics, 26*(2), 77-85.

Marcus, L. M., Kunce, L. J., & Schopler, E. (2005). Working with families. In F. Volkmar, R. Paul, A. Klin, & D. Cohen (Eds.), *Handbook of autism and pervasive developmental disorders* (3rd ed.; pp. 1055-1086). Hoboken, NJ: Wiley.

Martin, B. J., W., Logemann, J. A., Shaker, R., & Dodds, W. J. (1993). Normal laryngeal valving patterns during three breath-hold maneuvers: A pilot investigation. *Dysphagia, 8,* 11-20.

Martin, R. (1971). Catch them being good: Contingency contracting in the classroom. *Nation's Schools, 88*(5), 65-67.

Marzano, R. J., Pickering, D. J., & Pollock, J. E. (2001). *Classroom instruction that works: Research-based strategies for increasing student achievement.* Alexandria, VA: Association for Supervision and Curriculum Development.

Matson, J. L., Sevin, J. A., Fridley, D., & Love, S. R. (1990). Increasing spontaneous language in three autistic children. *Journal of Applied Behavior Analysis, 23,* 227-233.

McCarthy, M. P. (2003, October). Promoting problem-solving and self-evaluation in clinical education through a collaborative approach to supervision. *Perspectives on Administration and Supervision,* 20-26.

McCoy, K. (1995). *Teaching special learners in the general education classroom* (2nd ed.). Denver, CO: Love.

McEvoy, M., & Neilsen, S. (2001). Using functional behavioral assessment and functional communication training to assess and prevent challenging behavior. *Special Interest Division 12: Augmentative and Alternative Communication, 10*(1), 6-8.

McFarlane, S. (1988). Treatment of benign laryngeal disorders with traditional methods and techniques of voice therapy. *Ear, Nose, & Throat Journal, 67,* 425-435.

McFarlane, S., & Watterson, T. (1990). Vocal nodules: Endoscopic study of their variations and treatment. *Seminars in Speech and Language, 11*, 1.

McGee, G., Krantz, P. J., & McClannahan, L. E. (1985). The facilitative effects of incidental teaching on preposition use by autistic children. *Journal of Applied Behavior Analysis, 18*, 17–31.

McGee, G., Morrier, M., & Daly, T. (1999). An incidental teaching approach to early intervention for toddlers with autism. *Journal of the Association for Persons with Severe Handicaps, 24*, 133–146.

McLean, L., & Woods Cripe, J. (1997). The effectiveness of early intervention for children with communication disorders. In M. Guralnick (Ed.), *The effectiveness of early intervention* (pp. 349–429). Baltimore: Brookes.

McPherson, K. A., Kenny, D. J., Koheil, R., Bablish, K., Sochaniwskyj, A., & Milner, M. (1992). Ventilation and swallowing interactions of normal children and children with cerebral palsy. *Developmental Medicine and Child Neurology, 34*, 577–588.

McVeagh, P., Howman-Giles, R., & Kemp, A. (1987). Pulmonary aspiration studied by radionuclide milk scanning and barium swallow roentgenography. *American Journal of Diseases of Children, 141*(8), 917–921.

Merritt, D. D., & Culatta, B. (1998). *Language intervention in the classroom*. San Diego, CA: Singular.

Metsala, J., & Walley, A. (1998). Spoken vocabulary growth and the segmental restructuring of lexical representation: Precursors to phonemic awareness and early reading ability. In J. Metsala & L. Ehri (Eds.), *Word recognition in beginning literacy* (pp. 89–122). Mahwah, NJ: Erlbaum.

Meyers, S., & Woodford, L. (1992). *The fluency development system for young children*. Buffalo, NY: United Educational Services.

Miccio, A. W., & Ingrisano, D. (2000). The acquisition of fricatives and affricates: Evidence from a disordered phonological system. *American Journal of Speech-Language Pathology, 9*, 214–229.

Miller, J., & Paul, R. (1995). *The clinical assessment of language comprehension*. Baltimore: Brookes.

Miller, J. F., Long, S., McKinley, N., Thormann, S., Jones, M., & Nockerts, A. (2005). *Language sample analysis II: The Wisconsin guide*. Madison, WI: Wisconsin Department of Public Instruction.

Millikin, C. (1997). Symbol systems and vocabulary selection strategies. In S. Glennen & D. Decoste (Eds.), *Handbook on augmentative and alternative communication* (pp. 97–148). San Diego, CA: Singular.

Mirenda, P. (1997a). Functional communication training and augmentative communication: A research review. *Augmentative and Alternative Communication, 13*, 2007–225.

Mirenda, P. (1997b). Supporting individuals with challenging behavior through functional communication training and AAC: Research review. *Augmentative and Alternative Communication, 13*, 207–225.

Mirenda, P. (2003). Toward functional augmentative and alternative communication for students with autism: Manual signs, graphic symbols, and voice output communication aids. *Language, Speech, and Hearing Services in Schools, 34*, 202–215.

Miyamoto, R. T., Robbins, A. M., Osberger, M. J., Todd, S. L., Riley A. L., & Kirk, K. I. (1995). Comparison of multichannel tactile aids and multichannel cochlear implants in children with profound hearing impairments. *American Journal of Otology, 16*, 8–13.

Moeller, M. P. (1996, October). *Early intervention: Are we effective?* Paper presented at the Fourth International Symposium on Childhood Deafness, Kiawah Island, SC.

Moeller, M. P., Donaghy, K. F., Besuchaine, K. L., Lewis, D. E., & Stelmachowicz, P. G. (1996). Longitudinal study of FM system use in non-academic settings: Effects on language development. *Ear and Hearing, 17*, 28–41.

Moeller, M. P., & Luetke-Stahlman, B. (1990). Parents' use of Signing Exact English: A descriptive analysis. *Journal of Speech and Hearing Disorders, 55*, 327–338.

Moeller, M. P., & McConkey, A. J. (1983, November). *Evaluation of the hearing-impaired infant: What constitutes progress?* Miniseminar presented at the annual convention of the American Speech-Language-Hearing Association, Cincinnati, OH.

Moog, J., & Geers, A. (1985). EPIC: A program to accelerate academic progress in profoundly deaf children. *Volta Review, 87*, 259–277.

Moore, M., & Calvert, S. (2000). Brief report, Vocabulary acquisition for children with autism: Computer or teacher instruction. *Journal of Autism and Developmental Disabilities, 30*, 359–362.

Murry, T., & Woodson, G. (1992). Comparison of three methods for the management of vocal fold nodules. *Journal of Voice, 6*, 271–276.

Murry, T., & Woodson, G. (1995). Combined-modality treatment of adductor spasmodic dysphonia with botulium toxin and voice therapy. *Journal of Voice, 9*, 460–465.

National Reading Panel. (2000). *Teaching children to read: An evidence-based assessment of the scientific research literature on reading and its implications for reading instruction*. Washington, DC: National Institute of Child Health and Human Development. Retrieved February 3, 2007, from http://www.nationalreadingpanel.org/

National Research Council. (2001). *Education of children with autism*. Washington, DC: National Academy Press, Committee on Educational Interventions for Children with Autism, Division of Behavioral and Social Sciences and Education.

Nelson, K. E., Camarata, S. M., Welsh, J., Butkovsky, L., & Camarata, M. (1996). Conversational recasting treatment on the acquisition of grammar in children with specific language impairment and younger language normal children. *Journal of Speech, Language, and Hearing Research, 39*, 850–859.

Newman, L. A., Cleveland, R. H., Blickman, J. G., Hillman, R. E., & Jaramillo, D. (1991). Videofluoroscopic analysis of the infant swallow. *Investigative Radiology, 26*, 870–873.

Nilson, H., & Schneiderman, C. (1983). Classroom program for the prevention of vocal abuse and hoarseness in elementary school children. *Language, Speech, and Hearing Services in Schools, 14*, 121–127.

Nittrouer, S. (2002). From ear to cortex: A perspective on what clinicians need to understand about speech perception and language processing. *Language, Speech, and Hearing Services in Schools, 33*, 237–253.

No Child Left Behind Act. (2001). *Statement of purpose*. H.R.1-16 (9). Washington, DC: 107th Congress of the United States.

Norris, J. A., & Hoffman, P. R. (2005). Goals and targets: Facilitating the self-organization nature of a neuronetwork. In A. Kamhi & K. Pollock (Eds.), *Phonological disorders in children: Clinical decision making in assessment and intervention* (pp. 77–87). Baltimore: Brookes.

Odom, S., & Strain, P.(1984). Peer-mediated approaches to promoting children's social interaction: A review. *American Journal of Orthopsychiatry, 54*, 544–557.

Ohmae, Y., Logemann, J. A., Kaiser, P., Hanson, D. G., & Kahrilas, P. J. (1996). Effects of two breath-holding maneuvers on oropharyngeal swallow. *Annals of Otology, Rhinology, and Laryngology, 105*, 123–131.

Oke, N. J., & Schreibman, L. (1990). Training social initiations to a high-functioning autistic child: Assessment of collateral behavior change and generalization in a case study. *Journal of Autism and Developmental Disorders, 20*, 479–497.

Oller, K. (1978). Infant vocalization and the development of speech. *Allied Health and Behavior Sciences, 1*, 523–549.

Olswang, L., & Bain, B. (1991). Intervention issues for toddlers with specific language impairments. *Topics in Language Disorders, 11*, 69–86.

Onslow, M., Andrews, C., & Lincoln, M. (1994). A control/experimental trial of an operant treatment for early stuttering. *Journal of Speech and Hearing Research, 37*, 1244–1259.

Orlich, D. C. (1980). *Teaching strategies: A guide to better instruction*. Indianapolis, IN: D.C. Heath & Company.

Osberger, M. J., Maso, M., & Sam, L. K., (1993). Speech intelligibility of children with cochlear implants, tactile aids, or hearing aids. *Journal of Speech and Hearing Research, 36*, 186–203.

Osberger, M. J., Miyamoto, R. T., Zimmerman-Phillips, S., Kkemink, J. L., Stroer, B. S., Firszi, J. B., et al. (1991). Independent evaluation of the speech perception abilities of children with the Nucleus 22-channel cochlear implant sstem. *Ear and Hearing, 12*(4), 66S–80S.

Owens, R. (2004). *Language disorders: A functional approach to assessment and intervention* (4th ed.). Boston: Allyn & Bacon.

Panerai, S., Ferrante, L., & Zingale, M. (2002). Benefits of the Treatment and Education of Autistic and Communication Handicapped Children (TEACH) program as compared with non-specific approach. *Journal of Intellectual Disability Research, 46*, 318–327.

Parette, P., VanBiervliet, A., Reyna, J., & Heisserer, D. (Eds.). (1999). Families, culture and augmentative and alternative communication (AAS): A multimedia instructional program for related service personnel and family members. Retrieved July 7, 2003, from http://cstl.semo.edu/parette/homepage/database.pdf

Parsons, S., & Mitchell, P. (1999). What children with autism understand about thoughts and thought bubbles. *Autism, 3*, 17–38.

Paul, R. (2007). *Language disorders from infancy through adolescence: Assessment and intervention* (3rd ed.). St. Louis, MO: Mosby.

Paul, R., & Eldere, L. (2007). *The miniature guide to critical thinking concepts and tools* (4th ed.). Dillon Beach, CA: Foundation for Critical Thinking Press.

Peterson, S., Bonday, A., Vincent, Y., & Finnegan, C. (1995). Effect of altering communicative input for students with autism and non speech: Two case studies. *Augmentative and Alternative Communication, 11*, 93–100.

Pierce, K., & Shreibman, L. (1994). Teaching daily living skills to children with autism in unsupervised settings through pictorial self-management. *Journal of Applied Behavior Analysis, 27,* 471–482.

Pokorni, J. L., Worthington, C. K., & Jamison, P. J. (2004). Phonological awareness intervention: Comparison of Fast ForWord, Earobics, and LiPS. *Journal of Educational Research, 97,* 147–157.

Porzsolt, F., Ohletz, A., Gardner, D., Ruatti, H., Meier, H., Schlotz-Gorton, N., et al. (2003). Evidence-based decision making: The 6-step approach. *American College of Physicians Journal Club, 139*(3), 1–6.

Poteet, J. A., Choate, S., & Stewart, S. C. (1996). *Performance assessment and "special education" practices and prospects.* In E. Meyen, G. Vergason, & R. Whelan (Eds.), *Strategies for teaching exceptional children in inclusive settings* (pp. 209–242). Denver, CO: Love.

Pouderoux, P., & Kahrilas, P. J. (1995). Deglutive tongue force modulation by volition, volume, and viscosity in humans. *Gastroenterology, 108,* 1418–1426.

Prelock, P. (2007). *Treatment efficacy summary: Autistic spectrum disorders.* Rockville, MD: American Speech-Language-Hearing Association.

Prizant, B., & Wetherby, A. (1998). Understanding the continuum of discrete-trial traditional behavioral to social-pragmatic developmental approaches in communication enhancement for young children with autism/PDD. *Seminars in Speech and Language, 19,* 329–353.

Quist, R., & Lloyd, L. (1997). Principles and uses of technology. In L. Lloyd, D. Fuller, & H. Arvidson (Eds.), *Augmentative and alternative communication* (pp. 107–126). Boston: Allyn & Bacon.

Ramig, L. O., & Verdolini, K. (1998). Treatment efficacy: Voice disorders. *Journal of Speech, Language, and Hearing Research, 41,* 172–187.

Ramig, L. O., & Verdolini, K. (2007). *Treatment efficacy: Laryngeal-based voice disorders.* Rockville, MD: American Speech-Language-Hearing Association.

Rasley, A., Logemann, J. A., Kahrilas, P. J., Rademaker, A. W., Pauloski, B. R., & Dodds, W. J. (1993). Prevention of barium aspiration during videofluoroscopic swallowing studies. Value of change in posture. *AJR American Journal of Roentgenology, 160,* 1005–1009.

Ratclif, A., Caughlin,, S., & Lehman, M. (2002). Factors influencing ratings of speech naturalness in augmentative and alternative communication. *Augmentative and Alternative Communication 18*(1), 11–19.

Reed, V. A. (2005). *An introduction to children with language disorders.* Boston: Allyn & Bacon.

Reichle, J., & Wacker, D. (1993). *Communication alternatives to challenging behavior: Integrating functional assessment and intervention strategies.* Baltimore: Brookes.

Reinhartsen, D. B., Garfinkle, A. N., & Wolery, M. (2002). Engagement with toys in two-year-old children with autism: Teacher selection versus child choice. *Research and Practice for Persons with Severe Disabilities, 27,* 175–187.

Robbins, A. M., Osberger, M. J., Miyamoto, R. T., & Kessler, K. S. (1995). Language development in young children with cochlear implants. *Advances in Oto-Rhino-Laryngology, 50,* 160–165.

Robbins, J. A., & Levine, R. (1993). Swallowing after lateral medullary syndrome plus. *Clinics in Communication Disorders, 3,* 45–55.

Robey, R. R. (1998). A meta-analysis of clinical outcomes in the treatment of aphasia. *Journal of Speech, Language, and Hearing Research, 41,* 172–187.

Robey, R. R. (2004). A five-phase model for clinical-outcome research. *Journal of Communication Disorders, 5,* 401–411.

Robinson, L., & Owens, R. (1995). Functional augmentative communication and behavioral change. *Augmentative and Alternative Communication, 11,* 207–211.

Roehrig, S., Sutter, D., & Pierce, T. (2004, November). *An examination of passive oral motor exercises.* Poster presented at the annual convention of the American Speech-Language-Hearing Association, Philadelphia, PA.

Rogers, S. J., & Lewis, H. (1989). An effective day treatment model for young children with pervasive developmental disorders. *Journal of the American Academy of Child and Adolescent Psychiatry, 28,* 207–214.

Rogers, S. J. (1998). Neuropsychology of autism in young children and its implications for early intervention. *Mental Retardation and Developmental Disabilities Research Reviews, 4,* 104–112.

Rogers-Warren, A., & Warren, S. (1980). Mands for verbalization: Facilitating the generalization of newly trained language in children. *Behavior Modification, 4,* 230–245.

Roth, F., & Paul, R. (2007). Communication intervention principles. In R. Paul & C. W. Cascella (Eds.), *Introduction to clinical methods in communication disorders* (2nd ed., pp. 157–178). Baltimore: Brookes.

Roth, F. P., & Worthington, C. K. (1996). *Treatment resource manual.* San Diego, CA: Singular.

Roth, F., & Worthington, C. K. (2005). *Intervention resource manual for speech-language pathology* (3rd ed.). Clifton Park, NY: Appleton-Century-Crofts.

Rouse, C. E., & Kruger, A. B. (2004). Putting computerized instruction to the test: A randomized evaluation of a scientifically-based reading program. *Economics of Education Review, 23*, 323–338.

Roy, N., Bless, D., Helsey, D., & Ford, C. (1997). Manual circumlaryngeal therapy for functional dysphonia: An evaluation of short- and long-term treatment outcomes. *Journal of Voice, 11*(3), 321–331.

Roy, N., & Leeper, H. A. (1993). Effects of manual laryngeal musculoskeletal tension reduction technique as a treatment for functional voice disorders: Perceptual and acoustic measures. *Journal of Voice, 7*(3), 242–249.

Runyan, C., & Runyan, S. (1993). Therapy for school-age stutters: An update on the fluency rules program. In R. Curlee (Ed.), *Stuttering and related disorders of fluency* (pp. 101–114). New York: Thieme Medical.

Ryan, B., & Van Kirk Ryan, B. (1983). Programmed stuttering therapy for children: Comparisons of four establishment programs. *Journal of Fluency Disorders, 8*, 291–321.

Sabol, J. W., Lee, L., & Stempie, J. (1995). The value of vocal function exercises in the practice regimen of singers. *Journal of Voice, 9*, 27–36.

Sainato, D. M., Goldstein, H., & Strain, P. S. (1992). Effects on self-evaluation on preschool children's use of social interaction strategies with their classmates with autism. *Journal of Applied Behavior Analysis, 25*, 127–141.

Sarokoff, R. A., Taylor, B. A., & Poulson, C. I. (2001). Teaching children with autism to engage in conversational exchanges: Script fading with embedded textual stimuli. *Journal of Applied Behavior Analysis, 34*, 81–84.

Scherer, N., & Olswang, J. (1984). Role of mother's expansion in stimulating children's language production. *Journal of Speech and Hearing Research, 27*, 387–396.

Schlesinger, H., & Acree, M. (1984). Antecedents to achievement and adjustment in deaf adolescents: A longitudinal study of deaf children. In G. B. Anderson & D. Watson (Eds.), *The habilitation and rehabilitation of deaf adolescents* (pp. 48–61). Washington, DC: The National Academy of Gallaudet College.

Schlosser, R. W., McGhie-Richmond, D., Blacstien-Adler, S., Mirenda, P., Antonius, K., & Janzen, P. (2000). Training a school team to integrate technology meaningfully into the curriculum: Effects on student participation. *Journal of Special Education Technology, 15*, 31–44.

Schraeder, T. (2001, October). Three current hot issues related to professional ethics. *School-Based Issues, 2*(1), 28.

Schraeder, T. (2006). *School services in speech-language pathology.* Madison, WI: Pigwick Papers.

Schraeder, T. (2007). Professional performance review process for the school-based speech-language pathologist. *School-Based Issues, 8*(1), 3–6.

Schraeder, T., Quinn, M., Stockman, I., & Miller, J. (1999). Authentic assessment as an approach to speech-language screening, *American Journal of Speech-Language Pathology, 8*, 195–200.

Schwartz, I. S., Garfinkle, A., & Bauer, J. (1998). The Picture Exchange Communication System: Communicative outcomes for young children with disabilities. *Topics in Early Childhood Special Education, 18*, 144–159.

Shanahan, T. K., Logemann, J. A., Rademaker, A. W., Pauloski, B. R., & Kahrilas, P. J. (1993). Chin down posture effects on aspiration in dysphagic patients. *Archives of Physical Medicine and Rehabilitation, 74*, 736–739.

Shane, H. C., & Simmons, M. (2001, November). *Supports to enhance communication and improve problem behaviors.* Paper presented at the annual convention of the American Speech-Language-Hearing Association, New Orleans, LA.

Shearer, D. D., Kohler, F. W., Buchan, K. A., & McCullough, K. M. (1996). Promoting independent interactions between preschoolers with autism and their nondisabled peers: An analysis of self-monitoring. *Early Education and Development, 7*, 205–220.

Shelton, J. L., & Meyer, E. M. (1977). Catch them being good. *School Counselor, 25*(2), 110–115.

Shine, R. (1984). Assessment and fluency training with the young stutterers. In M. Peins (Ed.), *Contemporary approaches in stuttering therapy* (pp. 173–216). Boston: Little, Brown.

Shinn, M. R., & Hubbard. D. D. (1996). Curriculum-based measurement and problem-solving assessment: Basic procedures and outcomes. In E. Meyen, G. Vergason, & R. Whelan (Eds.), *Strategies for teaching exceptional children in inclusive settings* (pp. 243–278). Denver, CO: Love.

Shriberg, L. D. (1997). Developmental phonological disorders: One or many? In B. Hodson & M. Edwards (Eds.), *Perspectives in applied phonology* (pp. 105–127). Gaithersburg, MD: Aspen.

Sicotte, C., Lehoux, P., Fortier-Blanc, J., & Leblanc, Y. (2003). Feasibility and outcome evaluation of a telemedicine application in speech-language pathology. *Journal of Telemedicine and Telecare, 9*(5), 253-258.

Sigafoos, J. (1999). Creating opportunities for augmentative and alternative communication: Strategies for involving people with developmental disabilities. *Augmentative and Alternative Communication, 15*, 183-190.

Skinner, B. F. (1957). *Verbal behavior.* New York: Appleton-Century-Crofts.

Smith, S., & Thyme, K. (1976). Statistic research on changes in speech due to pedagologic treatment (the accent method). *Folia Phoniatricia, 28*, 98-103.

Soto, G., Huer, M., & Taylor, O. (1997). Multicultural issues. In L. Loyd, D. Fuller, & H. Arvidson (Eds.), *Augmentative and alternative communication* (pp. 406-413). Boston: Allyn & Bacon.

Starkweather, C., Gottwald, S., & Halfond, M. (1990). *Stuttering prevention: A clinical method.* Englewood Cliffs, NJ: Prentice-Hall.

Stempie, J. C., Lee, L., D'Amico, B., & Picup, B. (1994). Efficacy of vocal function exercises as a method of improving voice production. *Journal of Voice, 83*, 271-278.

Stitt, S., & Eger, D. (2006). *From evaluation to the ABCs of IEPs.* Retrieved April 1, 2007, from http://www.speechpathology.com

Strain, P. S., Kerr, M. M., & Ragland, E. U. (1979). Effects of peer mediated social initiation and prompting/reinforcement procedures on the social behaviors of autistic children. *Journal of Autism and Developmental Disorders, 9*, 41-54.

Strain, P. S., & Kohler, F. (1998). Peer-mediated social interventions for young children with autism. *Seminars in Speech and Language, 19*, 391-405.

Strong, C. J., & Clark, T. C. (1992). *Project SKI*HI outreach programming for hearing impaired infants and families: Recertification statement, questions, responses, and approval.* Washington, DC: Research in Education, Department of Education.

Strong, M., & Prinz, P. (1997). A study of the relationship between American Sign Language and English literacy. *Journal of Deaf Studies and Deaf Education, 2*, 37-46.

Swanson, H. L. (1996). Classification and dynamic assessment of children with learning disabilities. In E. Meyen, G. Vergason, & R. Whelan (Eds.), *Strategies for teaching exceptional children in inclusive settings* (pp. 191-208). Denver, CO: Love.

Swanson, L., Fey, M., Mills, C., & Hood, S. (2005). Use of narrative based language intervention with children who have specific language impairment.

American Journal of Speech-Language Pathology, 14, 131-141.

Swengel, K., & Marquette, J. (1997). Service delivery in AAC. In S. Glennen & D. Decoste (Eds.), *Handbook of augmentative and alternative communication* (pp. 21-57). San Diego, CA: Singular.

Szeto, A., Allen, E., & Littrell, M. (1993). Comparison of speech and accuracy for selected electronic communication devices and input methods. *Augmentative and Alternative Communication, 9*, 229-242.

Taylor, B. A., Levin L., & Jasper, S. (1999). Increasing play-related statements in children with autism toward their siblings: Effects of video modeling. *Journal of Developmental and Physical Disabilities, 11*, 253-264.

Tessmer, M., & Harris, D. (1992). *Analyzing the instructional setting: Environmental analysis.* London: Kogan Page.

Thiemann, K., & Goldstein, H. (2004). Effects of peer training and written-text cuing on social communication of school-age children with pervasive developmental disorder. *Journal of Speech, Language, and Hearing Research, 47*, 126-144.

Tibbets, D. F. (1995). *Language intervention beyond the primary grades for clinicians by clinicians.* Austin, TX: Pro-Ed.

Ticanci, M. (2004). Comparing the Picture Exchange Communication System and sign language training for children with autism. *Focus on Autism and Other Developmental Disabilities, 19*, 152-163.

Tobey, E., Geers, A. E., & Brenner, C. (1994). Speech production results: Speech feature acquisition. *Volta Review, 96*, 109-129.

Tolia, V., Kuhns, L., & Kauffman, R. (1993). Correlation of gastric emptying at one and two hours following formula feeding. *Pediatric Radiology, 23*, 26-28.

Tye-Murray, N., Spencer, L., & Woodworth, G. G. (1995). Acquisition of speech by children who have prolonged cochlear implant experience. *Journal of Speech and Hearing Research, 38*, 327-338.

Tyler, A. (2005). Planning and monitoring intervention programs. In A. Kamhi & K. Pollock (Eds.), *Phonological disorders in children: Clinical decision making in assessment and intervention* (pp. 123-137). Baltimore: Brookes.

Tyler, A., Lewis, K., Haskill, A., & Tolbert, L. (2003). Efficacy of cross-domain effects of a morphosyntax and a phonologic intervention. *Language, Speech, and Hearing Services in Schools, 33*, 52-66.

Tyler, A., & Sandoval, K. (1994). Preschoolers with phonological and language disorders: Treating different linguistic domains. *Language, Speech, and Hearing Services in Schools, 25,* 215-234.

U.S. Department of Education. (2000). *22nd annual report to Congress on the implementation of the Individuals with Disabilities Education Act (IDEA)*, Washington, DC: U.S. Government Printing Office.

U.S. Preventive Services Task Force. (1989) [Electronic version]. Evaluating and ranking research evidence. Retrieved February 3, 2007, from http://www.ahrq.gov

Van Riper, C., & Emerick, L. (1984). *Speech correction: An introduction to speech pathology and audiology* (7th ed.). Englewood Cliffs, NJ: Prentice-Hall.

Veis, S., Logemann, J. A., & Colangelo, L. (1997, November). *Effects of three techniques on tongue base posterior movement.* Paper presented at the annual convention of the American Speech-Language-Hearing Association, Boston.

Velleman, S., & Vihman, M. (2002). Whole-word phonology and templates: Trap, bootstrap, or some of each? *Language, Speech, and Hearing Services in Schools, 33,* 9-24.

Venkatagiri, H. (1993). Efficiency of lexical prediction as a communication acceleration technique. *Augmentative and Alternative Communication, 12,* 126-134.

Vennkatagiri, H. (1999). Efficient keyboard layouts for sequential access in augmentative and alternative communication. *Augmentative and Alternative Communication, 15,* 126-134.

Verdolini-Marston, K., Burk, M., Lessac, A., Glaze, L., & Caldwell, E. (1995). Preliminary study of two methods of treatment for laryngeal nodules. *Journal of Voice, 9,* 74-85.

Verdolini-Marston, K., Sandage, M., & Titze, I. (1994). Effect of hydration treatments on laryngeal nodules and polyps and related voice measures. *Journal of Voice, 8,* 30-47.

Vihman, M. (2004). Later phonological development. In J. Bernthal & N. Bankson (Eds.), *Articulation and phonological disorders* (5th ed., pp. 105-138). Boston: Allyn & Bacon.

Villa, R. A., & Thousand, J. S. (1995). *Creating an inclusive school.* Alexandria, VA: Association for Supervision and Curriculum Development.

Walley, A., Metsala, J., & Garlock, V. (2003). Spoken vocabulary growth: Its role in the development of phoneme awareness and early reading ability. *Reading and Writing: An Interdisciplinary Journal, 16,* 5-20.

Warner, J., & Bryan, C. (1995). *The unauthorized teacher's survival guide.* Indianapolis, IN: Park Avenue Publications.

Warren, S. (1991). Enhancing communication and language development with milieu teaching procedures. In E. Cipani (Ed.), *A guide to developing language competence in preschool children with severe and moderate handicaps* (pp. 68-93). Springfield, IL: Charles C Thomas.

Warren, S. E., & Kaiser, A. P. (1986). Incidental language teaching: A critical review. *Journal of Speech and Hearing Disorders, 51,* 291-299.

Watanabe, M., & Sturmey, P. (2003). The effect of choice-making opportunities during activity schedules on task engagement of adults with autism. *Journal of Autism and Developmental Disorders, 33,* 535-538.

Watkins, S. (1987). Long-term effects of home intervention with hearing impaired children. *American Annals of the Deaf, 132,* 267-271.

Watterson, T., Hansen-Magorian, H., & McFarlane, S. C. (1990). A demographic description of laryngeal contact ulcer patients. *Journal of Voice, 4,* 71-75.

Weber, F., Wooldridge, M., & Baum, J. (1986). An ultrasonographic study of the organization of sucking and swallowing by newborn infants. *Developmental Medicine and Child Neurology, 28,* 19-24.

Webne-Behrman, H. (2005). *Eight steps for conflict resolution.* Retrieved April 16, 2007, from http://www.ohrd.wisc.edu/onlinetraining/resolution/index.asp

Weismer, S. E., & Evans, J. (2002). The role of processing imitations in early identification of specific language impairments. *Topics in Language Disorders, 22,* 15-29.

Weismer, S., & Hesketh, L. (1993). The influence of prosodic and gestural cues on novel word acquisition by children with specific language impairment. *Journal of Speech and Hearing Research, 36,* 1013-1025.

Weismer, S. E., & Robertson, S. (2006). Focused stimulation approach to language intervention. In R. McCauley & M. Fey (Eds.), *Treatment of language disorders in children* (pp. 175-202). Baltimore: Brookes.

Weismer, S. E., & Schraeder, T. (1993). Discourse characteristics and verbal reasoning: wait time effects on the performance of children with language learning disabilities. *Exceptional Education Canada, 3*(3), 71-92.

Wellman, H., Baron-Cohen, S., Caswell, R., Gomez, J. C., Swettenham, J., Toye, E., et al. (2002). Thought bubbles help children with autism acquire an alternative to theory of mind. *Autism, 6,* 343-363.

Wendt, O., Schlosser, R., & Lloyd, L. (2004, November). *AAC for children with autism: A meta-analysis of intervention outcomes.* Paper presented at the annual convention of the American Speech-Language-Hearing Association, Philadelphia.

Wesson, C. L., & King, R. P. (1996). Portfolio assessment and special education students. In E. Meyen, G. Vergason, & R. Whelan (Eds.), *Strategies for teaching exceptional children in inclusive settings.* (pp. 293–303). Denver, CO: Love.

Westling, D., & Fox, L. (2000). *Teaching students with severe disabilities* (2nd ed.). Upper Saddle River, NJ: Merrill.

Weston, A., & Bain, B. (2003, November). *Current versus evidence-based practice in phonological intervention: A dilemma.* Poster session presented at the annual convention of the American Speech-Language-Hearing Association, Chicago.

Whalon, C., & Schreibman, L. (2003). Joint attention training for children with autism using behavior modification procedures. *Journal of Child Psychology and Psychiatry, 44,* 456–468.

White, P. (2004). *Managing threatening confrontations.* Verona, WI: Attainment Company.

White, S. (1984). *Antecedents of language functioning in the deaf: Implications for early intervention. Project summary.* Washington, DC: U.S. Department of Education.

Wilkinson, K., & McIlvane, W. (2002). Considerations in teaching graphic symbols to beginning communicators. In J. Reichle, D. Beukelman, & J. Light (Eds.), *Exemplary practices for beginning communicators: Implications for AAC* (pp. 273–321). Baltimore: Brookes.

Williams, A. (2005). From developmental norms to distance metrics: Past, present, and future directions for target selection practices. In A. Kamhi & K. Pollock (Eds.), *Phonological disorders in children: Clinical decision making in assessment and intervention* (pp. 101–108). Baltimore: Brookes.

Willging, J. P. (2000). Benefit of feeding assessment before pediatric airway reconstruction. *Laryngoscope, 110,* 825–834.

Wisconsin Department of Public Instruction. (2004). *Student records and confidentiality.* Madison, WI: Department of Public Instruction.

Yamaguchi, H., Hotsukura, Y., Konda, R., Hanyuu, Y., Horiguchi, S., Imaizumi, S., et al. (1986). Nonsurgical therapy for vocal nodules. *Folia Phoniatrica, 38,* 372–373.

Yamamoto, J., & Miya, M. (1999). Acquisition and trans-fer of sentence construction in autistic students: Analysis by computer-based teaching. *Research in Developmental Disabilities, 20,* 355–377.

Yamashita, J. (2003). Processes of taking a gap-filling test: Comparison of skilled and less skilled EFL readers. *Language Testing, 20*(3), 267–293.

Yang, W. T., Loveday, E. J., Metrewell, C., & Sullivean, P. B. (1997). Ultrasound assessment of swallowing in malnourished disabled children. *British Journal of Radiology, 70,* 992–994.

Yaruss, J. S., Quesal, R. W., Reeves, L., Molt, L., Kluetz, B., Caruso, A. J., et al. (2002). Speech treatment and support group experiences of people who participate in the National Stuttering Association. *Journal of Fluency Disorders, 27,* 115–135.

Yeargin-Allsopp, M., Rice, C., Karapurkar, T., Doernberg, N., Boyle, C., & Murphy, C. (2003). Prevalence of autism in a US metropolitan area. *Journal of the American Medical Association, 289,* 49–55.

Ylvisaker, M. & Logemann, J. A. (1998). Therapy for feeding and swallowing head injury. In M. Ylvisaker (Ed.) *Traumatic brain injury rehabilitation: children and adolescents* (2nd ed, pp 85–99). Boston: Butterworth-Heinemann.

Yoder, P. J., & Layton, T. L. (1988). Speech following sign language training in autistic children with minimal verbal language. *Journal of Autism and Developmental Disorders, 18,* 217–230.

Yoder, P., & Stone, W. (2006). Randomized comparison of two communication interventions for preschoolers with autism spectrum disorders. *Journal of Consulting and Clinical Psychology, 74*(3), 426–435.

Yoder, P., Spruytenburg, H., Edwards, A., & Davies, B. (1995). Effects of verbal routine contexts and expansions on gains in the mean length of utterance of children with developmental delays. *Language Speech and Hearing Services in Schools, 26,* 21–32.

Yoder, P., Warren, S., Kim, K., & Gazdag, G. (1994). Facilitating prelinguistic communication skills in young children with developmental delay. *Journal of Speech and Hearing Research, 37,* 841–851.

Zangari, C., & Kangas, K. (1997). Intervention principles and procedures. In L. Lloyd, D. Fuller, & H. Arvidson (Eds.), *Augmentative and alternative communication* (pp. 235–253). Boston: Allyn & Bacon.

Zwitman, D. H., & Calcaterra, T. C. (1973). The "silent cough" method for vocal hyperfunction. *Journal of Speech and Hearing Disorders, 38*(1), 119–125.

APPENDIX 5–1

Useful Web-Based Resources

Bandolier—A U.K.-based resource for a wide range of information on aspects of health care services from an evidence-based perspective. http://www.jr2.ox.ac.uk/bandolier

British Medical Journal—Provides all articles published since 1994 to be viewed online; journal may be searched by subject or author. http://www.bmj.com

Campbell Collaboration—Publishes guidelines for public policy and clinical practice. http://www.campbellcollaboration.org

Cochrane Collaboration—Publishes guidelines for public policy and clinical practice. http://www.cochrane.org

Compendium of EBP [Evidence-Based Practice] Guidelines and Systematic Reviews—Established by the American Speech-Language-Hearing Association (ASHA) to assess the quality of professional literature. http://www.asha.org/members/ebp/compendium

ERIC—A database administered by the U.S. National Library of Education; it provides bibliographic information about journal articles and other publications in the field of education and related disciplines; it includes worldwide coverage. http://askeric.org/Eric

U.S. Economic & Social Research Council (ESRC) Evidence Network—A program funded by the Economic and Social Research Council; the site contains a wide variety of material on evidence-based policy and practice in the social sciences, including a list of research databases. http://www.evidencenetwork.org

Google Scholar—A search engine that sorts articles the way researchers do, weighing the full text of each article, the author, the publication in which the article appears, and how often the piece has been cited in other literature. http://www.scholar.google.com

Joseph Rowntree Foundation—Provides summaries of all studies funded by this U.K.-based Foundation through its "Findings" series. http://www.jrf.org.uk

Making Research Count—This national initiative from the United Kingdom provides a bridge between social care practice and research; also provides research-based support to persons working in the personal social services and the National Health Service (NHS) across adult and children's services. http://www.uea.ac.uk/swk/research/mrc/welcome.htm

Medline—Focuses on health-related issues; available to the general public at no cost. http://www.MEDLINE.com

National Reading Panel (NRP)—Summarizes the available evidence on interventions and instruction supporting reading in five areas: vocabulary, fluency, phonemic awareness, comprehension, and phonics; the NRP report is available at no cost at http://www.nationalreadingpanel.org

Research Informed Practice Site—Includes downloadable summaries of research, including some appraisals of research; a U.K.-based site designed for busy education practitioners. http://www.standards.dfes.gov.uk/research

Research in Practice—An organization funded by the U.K.'s national Department of Health/Association of Directors of Social Services, set up to promote evidence-based practice in social care; provides searchable evidence including summaries (brief appraisals) of key reviews. http://www.rip.org.uk

Resource Discovery Network (RDN) Virtual Training Suite—A U.K.-based Internet gateway for the social sciences; provides guides to the conduct of research using the Internet, including one for social workers. http://www.vts.rdn.ac.uk/tutorial/social-worker

Social Care Institute for Excellence (SCIE)—Provides access to the U.K.'s national electronic Library of Social Care (eLC), which includes Care-Data, a searchable database of social care abstracts. http://www.sci.org.uk

Social Policy Research Unit—Provides details of studies conducted in the related fields of social security, social care, and health care, with many studies concerned with disabilities; located at York University. http://www.york.ac.uk/inst/spru/pubs/researchwks.htm

Turning Research into Practice (TRIP)—Searches more than 55 websites of high-quality evidence-based health information such as the professional journals. http://www.tripdatabase.com

U.S. Department of Health and Human Services' Agency for Healthcare Research and Quality—A resource for evidence-based practice guidelines and regular updates and summaries of clinical outcomes research related to health care. http://www.ahrq.gov

U.S. Preventive Services Task Force (USP-STF)—Oversees systematic reviews of effectiveness evidence and publishes guidelines that may be useful to both speech-language pathologists and audiologists working with children and youth. http://www.ahrq.gov/clinic/uspstf/uspsnbhr.htm

What Works Clearinghouse of the U.S. Department of Education's Institute of Education Sciences (IES)—Provides systematic reports on educational interventions, including intervention reports. http://www.w-w-c.org

Chapter 6
PROBLEM BEHAVIOR MANAGEMENT AND CONFLICT RESOLUTION

RELATED VOCABULARY

assertive communication Conveying one's needs and concerns clearly and specifically while respecting the needs of the other party.

BATNA The *b*est *a*lternative *t*o a *n*egotiated *a*greement.

foreshadowing Providing the expected outcome or a verbal description of what is expected to happen.

forced choice Limiting a student's choices to that between two outcomes that both are acceptable to the learning process or appropriate to the educational environment.

intrinsic motivation Self-driven desire or drive devoid of any outside influences.

MLATNA The *m*ost *l*ikely *a*lternative *t*o a *n*egotiated *a*greement.

respite care Short-term care provided so that long-term caregivers may have a break from their ongoing duties.

self-regulation The ability to control one's own emotions.

stigma A mark of discredit or disgrace.

tactile defensiveness Hypersensitive reaction to touch or texture.

WATNA The *w*orst *a*lternative *t*o a *n*egotiated *a*greement.

Introduction

The school-based speech-language pathologist (SLP) is immersed in a people-oriented profession. Strategies for dealing with conflict are needed. Conflict may arise in various types of interactions, including (1) student-to-student, (2) student-to-SLP, (3) parent-to-student, (4) SLP-to-parent, and (5) professional-to-SLP. It is estimated that 15% to 20% of school-aged children in the United States exhibit behavior problems and that 1% and 5% of those students have severe behavior problems. Behavior problems often are rooted in inadequate communication skills. Carr and colleagues (1994) provided extensive research showing that problem behaviors serve a purpose for those exhibiting it and that communication intervention is effective. The following examples demonstrate how an inability to express a need may result in undesirable behaviors.

- A student standing in the lunch line pushes another student because of an inability to express a need for more physical space.
- A student frustrated by an academic challenge acts out as a way of escaping the challenge.
- A student with an inability to understand directions appears noncompliant.
- A student has an unmet physical need and cannot attend to the language of the lesson until that physical need is met.
- A student is unable to attend to the language of a lesson because of an obsessive-compulsive disorder, oppositional defiant disorder, anxiety disorder, attention deficit/hyperactivity disorder, the sequelae of fetal alcohol syndrome, a sensory deficit, or **tactile defensiveness**.
- A student cannot attend to the language of the lesson because of emotional turmoil related to home and family issues.
- A student has not yet developed adequate cause-and-effect reasoning.

- A student acts out because of behavioral patterns that have developed in the home environment.

Olson (2007) identified five reasons why students with language disorders often exhibit other educational needs in the areas of behavior and social skills. Olson's work can be summarized as follows: (1) challenges with cooperative learning or play group formats (Brinton, Fujiki, & Higbee, 1998; Brinton, Fujiki, Montague, & Hanton, 2000; Fujiki, Brinton, Isaacson, & Summers, 2001; Fukiki, Brinton, Hart, & Fitzgerald, 1999; Nungesser & Watkins, 2005); (2) learning inhibited by aggressive behaviors (Fujiki, Brinton, & Clarke, 2002; Fujiki, Spackman, Brinton, & Hall, 2004; Johnston & Reichle, 1993); (3) feelings or needs expressed with inappropriate behaviors (Johnston & Reichle, 1993; Nungesser & Watkins, 2005); (4) social withdrawal (Fujiki et al., 2001; Nungesser & Watkins, 2005; Redmond & Rice, 1998); and (5) rejection by classmates (Brinton et al., 2000). Many children in America do not experience happy, safe childhoods. It is estimated that 13 million children live in poverty; 9 million children lack health insurance; more than 6 million children are left home alone after school each day; almost 900,000 children each year are victims of abuse or neglect; and one American child or teen is killed by gunfire approximately every three hours (Children's Defense Fund, 2005). Children who face these challenging life situations may act out as a way of coping with the stress. Dealing with problem behaviors is a complex task because the potential causes are so many and so varied.

Whatever the cause of the undesirable behavior, Hegde and Davis (1995) recommended response reduction strategies, which may be either direct or indirect. With the direct response reduction strategy, use of a contingency that reduces the occurrence of the undesirable behavior is required. This teaches the child what not to do. With the indirect strategy, a contingency is placed on a desirable behavior. When the desirable behavior increases, it will have an indirect effect of decreasing the undesirable behavior. The indirect strategy not only teaches the child what not to do but also identifies what to do instead.

Prior, Proper Planning and Proactive Strategies

Whatever the cause of the unacceptable behaviors exhibited by a child, the SLP must know and use conflict resolution strategies just as readily as he or she must know and use clinical strategies. Canter and Canter (1985) offered some proactive strategies that are applicable to all age groups. First, the SLP must establish clear expectations. This is accomplished by developing and posting a discipline plan in the educational environment. The plan should consist of no more than three to five rules, the rewards for following those rules, and the consequences for what happens when the rules are not followed. Picture symbols, accompanied by the printed words, may be used for young students who have not yet learned to read as well as for older students who struggle with literacy. The rules should be stated in a positive, rather than punitive, manner: For example, the SLP can say, "Use your walking feet," instead of "Don't run in the halls." The rules also should be stated in specific language: The SLP can say, "Keep hands, feet, and objects to yourself," instead of "Don't be naughty." The rewards and consequences must be meaningful for the students. If the students do not feel any **intrinsic motivation** regarding the rewards or consequences, compliance with the rules is unlikely. Motivation can be provided in various ways, as seen in the following scenarios from real-life clinical practice:

- An SLP reported that her elementary students had grown tired of stickers and no longer found them rewarding. Yet they were delighted when she shared her hand sanitizer gel. This SLP offered a pump from her hand sanitizer gel as a tangible reward for on-task behaviors. The students honored the rules she had established, and germs were kept to a minimum during the flu season.
- Another SLP discovered that a phone call home to a parent was highly motivating for a sixth grade student. This was an example of how an activity that sometimes is used as a negative consequence also could be used as a reward.
- Another school-based SLP reported that one of the most popular rewards among her students was allowing an older child the privilege of teaching younger children a speech-language game after a set number of reward points had been earned. Students often enjoy teaching others "fun" learning activities.
- Another SLP reported that an unruly student complied with rules if he was given a blank sheet of paper at the end of the day. He kept his "important papers" in a professional-looking briefcase that he carried with him at all times.

Finding the tangible reward that is highly motivating requires creativity and an understanding of each student's unique personality. Rewards do not always need to be tangible. In general, it is best to start out with verbal praise or social rewards. If that is sufficient, then imposing tangible rewards is unnecessary. If tangible rewards are not enough, however, then edible reinforcements may be tried as a last resort.

Students must actually be taught the rules, rewards, and consequences. Simply posting them is not sufficient. Role-playing sessions, demonstrations of rewards and consequences, question-and-answer sessions, video clips followed by guided questions, and periodic reviews are powerful tools that help students increase and retain their understanding. Semantic mapping may help the students comprehend positive and negative outcomes. Cause-and-effect discussions also are valuable. Social stories are another way in which students may gain a deeper meaning of the rules, rewards, and consequences. Application of the rules, rewards, and consequences must be consistent. If students believe the potential consequences are just a bluff, with no actual follow-through, their intrinsic motivation for honoring the rules will be diminished. Conversely, if they believe they were not given a reward that was promised, their trust level will be diminished and rapport will be seriously compromised.

A positive feeling tone should always be the focus. Verbal praise for on-task behaviors is just as important as corrective feedback for off-task behaviors. Verbal praise and "do" statements help students learn what behaviors are expected of them. Whenever possible, the SLP should follow a negative directive with a positive comment as soon as possible. In the following example, the SLP uses this approach to correct a student who is demonstrating unsafe behavior:

> SLP: You need to keep your bottom on your chair and your feet on the floor so that you will be safe.
>
> *Student sits down and stops rocking the chair.*
>
> SLP: Thank you for sitting safely. Now we can continue learning and not worry about an accident.

In this instance, a clear expectation is given in direct language. After the student complies, the compliance is acknowledged and a rationale is provided. The positive verbal praise was earned and acknowledged.

Foreshadowing expectations gives students a clear understanding of what they should do in the upcoming task or event. For example, before leaving a classroom, the SLP bends down to the child's level, smiles, and says, "We're going back to the classroom. I will hold your hand. We will use our walking feet and our quiet voices as we walk back to your room."

It is essential that the school principal and administrative personnel in charge of discipline issues be aware of the rules, rewards, and consequences that the SLP has established. Doing so ensures administrative support when conflicts arise. Conversely, the SLP should participate in the same discipline-related inservice training with other educators. The SLP must be part of the whole school team that enforces the school discipline policies and procedures consistently throughout the building. The entire school climate is affected by the discipline plan and philosophy.

Parents, caregivers, and legal guardians must be made aware of the rules, rewards, and consequences. If the parents are aware of the rules, rewards, and consequences before they are enforced, their support at times of infraction may be stronger. The first contact with the parents should be a positive one. For example, a good news phone call or note home during the first week of class may help establish a positive, cooperative feeling tone. Establishing a positive home-school partnership first will make it easier if a need to discuss negative issues arises later on.

Designing the learning environment for success is an important proactive strategy. For example, having the classroom wastebasket, pencil sharpener, tissue box, sink, supplies, and student work cubbies all in one small congested area creates an environment ripe for conflict. It forces the students to be in close proximity to one another. Close proximity makes it harder for students to keep their hands, feet, and objects to themselves. If possible, such items should be located in different areas of the room so that congestion is kept to a minimum. Walkways and doorways should be kept clear. Students who have chronic behavioral issues should be positioned so that other students with more compliant behaviors surround them. Peer models are very powerful. Positioning the student who wants control, who seeks attention, who is an underachiever, or who appears hostile in a far corner of the room, away from peers, only alienates that student and invites more acting-out behaviors as the child seeks attention. Keeping the child close to the learning action and showering him or her with positive praise for on-task behaviors may establish a pathway for compliance.

Using proactive strategies and having a plan in place for conflict resolution will help the SLP remain calm and focused in the face of unacceptable student behaviors. When a student expresses hostility, it is important for the SLP to acknowledge the student's feeling, as in the following example:

> SLP: It's time to review your vocabulary flashcards.
>
> STUDENT: I hate this dumb, stupid stuff.
>
> SLP: You don't like doing your vocabulary flashcards. It's hard work. The more you do them, the easier it will get. After you finish your vocabulary work, you can have some time on the computer.

Another way to deal with hostile behavior is by giving the student a **forced choice**:

SLP: It's time to review your vocabulary flashcards.

STUDENT: I hate this dumb, stupid stuff.

SLP: You have a choice. You may review your vocabulary flashcards with me at this table, or we can go back to your desk and review them there.

The SLP must be knowledgeable about typical child and adolescent development. For example, the SLP may need to divide a 40-minute session into four 10-minute activities for the 4-year-old child. The typical attention span for that age level is 7 to 15 minutes. The SLP may need to use the same strategy with a middle school student who demonstrates the cognitive abilities of a younger child. Likewise, the SLP must know the sleeping patterns and eating patterns of the preschooler. Scheduling an articulation session during nap time is not wise and will not yield optimum performance. In addition, the SLP must know the side effects of the medications that students have been prescribed. The student who is experiencing chronic dry mouth as a side effect of a medication may exhibit noncompliant behaviors because he or she needs a drink of water.

Whenever dealing with a noncompliant behavior, the SLP needs to consider the purpose that the behavior serves. Providing an older student with a rationale for the behavioral expectation and involving him or her in the decision-making process will help foster a positive, cooperative feeling tone. Robl offers these words of wisdom:

Flexibility is one issue that Richard Lavoie nicely summed up when he said that no student with learning disabilities should ever have a good day, because then his or her teachers think that he or she can perform to that ability level every day. This is also true of behavior. We need to be flexible. Kids have days when they can keep behaviors under control and days when they need more assistance. Off-task behaviors tend to become more prevalent during unstructured, unsupervised transition and less prevalent when students are assisted with self-regulation. When a kindergarten class moves from a group communication circle time while seated on the floor to the next activity that will be conducted at tables, the SLP is wise to have the students make the transition in small groups, rather than all at once. For example: "All those students wearing the color red may go to the table; now those students whose names begin with the letter T may go to the table; now anyone wearing glasses may go" [and so on]. (G. Robl, personal communication, June 22, 2005)

Establishing a safe environment is a proactive strategy that is important at all grade levels. Warner and Bryan (1995) offered some measures to help prevent thefts on school campuses. Warner and Bryan's recommendations are summarized here:

- Tell students not to bring valuable items to school.
- Keep your purse, identification, and money locked up.
- Be vigilant of student behaviors in unstructured settings.
- Do not leave any valuable items in school overnight.
- Do not leave valuables in a vehicle.
- Tell students not to leave valuables in their lockers.
- Do not allow students to go through another person's belongings.
- Prohibit students from selling items to each other at school.

White (2004) recommended that SLPs, educators, parents, and caregivers examine their attitudes regarding the student's challenging behaviors. White encouraged responsible adults to reframe attitudes in terms of behavioral challenges rather than behavioral problems. Professionals must accept the behavioral challenge as part of the student's disability. The challenge belongs to the professional. The behavioral resolution must be individualized, least restrictive, proactive, and not impose a **stigma** on the child. White recommended a team approach so that no one professional, parent, or caregiver experiences burnout. The parents or caregivers need a **respite care** plan, and school professionals need to work together. The team approach must be person centered. The team must analyze the communicative intent of the behaviors. How is the current unacceptable behavior meeting the child's needs? What pressures are causing or stimulating the behavior? The team must analyze the child's environment and consider changes in the environment before considering changes in the person. The environment must be modified so that the negative precipitating factors are minimized and opportunities for enrichment and growth are maximized.

The team must increase communications and positive interactions with the student during non-crisis times and foster independence rather than interdependence. Any feedback needs to be within the individual student's sphere of comprehension. Sometimes visual cues are needed to help the student understand the feedback; for example, the SLP may reinforce statements by holding up cardboard disks of different colors. If the student's behavior is acceptable, the SLP holds up a green disk which means on-task, acceptable behaviors. If the student's behavior is irritating another individual, the SLP holds up a yellow disk which means irritating behaviors. Finally, if the student's behavior is not appropriate, the SLP holds up a red disk which means unacceptable behaviors that must stop. Humor, diversions, and physical exercise should be considered as proactive strategies. The behavior plan should be written into the IEP so that all of the involved parties are consistent in their approach, and so that parents or legal guardians can approve the plan.

Creating a Culture of Community

Perhaps the most effective, yet most difficult proactive strategy is to move beyond the realm of discipline into the realm of establishing a classroom community. Kohn (1996) pointed out that taking time to teach children to care about each other also may have a positive influence on their enthusiasm for learning academic material. Students need to feel safe in order to take intellectual risks. They need to feel comfortable before they can pur-

posefully tackle challenges that make them feel uncomfortable. The fear of being judged or humiliated has a detrimental effect on the learning process. Academic excellence may be achieved only if children have positive feelings about school, the school environment, and each other.

Johnson and Johnson (1995) described approaches to discipline on a continuum and the costs and benefits of using each type of program. At one end of the continuum are programs based on adult-administered external rewards and punishments. These types of programs are designed with the idea that faculty members control and manage student behavior. At the other end of the continuum are discipline programs that focus on teaching students the competencies and skills they need so that they can manage their own behaviors. These types of programs are designed to teach peer mediation skills so that students may self-regulate their behaviors.

Most discipline programs are clustered at the external rewards-punishments end of the continuum. Programs that use external rewards and punishments are costly because students must be continuously observed and authority figures are required to resolve conflicts. They encourage a "don't-get-caught" attitude in the minds of students, rather than development of a sense of personal responsibility. Students are not empowered by external rewards and punishments. Schools that use an external rewards-punishments system may achieve an orderly learning environment, but such systems do not help students learn the conflict resolution skills and attitudes they need to become productive citizens.

Programs at the other end of the continuum teach **self-regulation**. Students learn to monitor a situation, assess interactive behaviors, and take another person's perspective into consideration. Learning self-regulation advances their cognitive and social development. Students are given opportunities to make decisions and reflect on those decisions. When students learn self-regulation, educators are able to focus on instruction, rather than on control. Teaching self-regulation, however, also is very time-consuming and often requires one-on-one discussions with guided questions. Self-regulation does not simply spring from within; rather, it must be taught through example, explanation, model imitation, metacognitive processing, self-reflection, and behavior management procedures such as those offered by Hegde and Davis (1995).

Curwin and Mendler (1999) pointed out that most students are able to follow a social contract that the entire class has created. Some students, however, must have an individual contract in order to comply with social norms. The SLP who uses inclusive practices must be involved with general educators to implement a proactive discipline program. Curwin and Mendler described eight positive strategies for dealing with confrontational students who require individualized behavioral contracts: positive student confrontation; family intervention; comprehensive social contract; cognitive behavior modification; role reversal; videotaping; audiotaping; and using older students as resources. These strategies are described next.

Positive Student Confrontation

Positive confrontation involves setting aside some time to meet individually with the student and attempting to resolve differences through negotiation. It requires the SLP to be willing to share directly with the student, to take the risk of hearing unpleasant things from that student, and to consider program modifications for the student. The SLP begins by describing the problem, the process, and his or her role. (*Example*: "I'm here to see if I can help you find a way to settle down your behaviors so that I can teach and you can learn.") Then the SLP and the student share feelings of dislike, resentment, anger, or frustration. (*Example*: "Tell me what makes you so angry. Then I'll tell you what makes me angry.") Each party must paraphrase what he or she hears from the other. Next, the SLP and the student share appreciations. (*Example*: "This is what I like about you . . . ") Again, each party must paraphrase what he or she hears from the other. Then the SLP and the student make demands. (*Example*: "Tell me what you want to be different.") Then the SLP and the student negotiate a solution. (*Example*: "Tell me what you're willing to do differently.") Once an agreement is reached, the plan is put in

writing and signed by both parties. A follow-up meeting is scheduled. The student and the SLP both look forward to the follow-up meeting to discuss how well it has worked and how each party feels about it.

Family Intervention

In family intervention, the SLP meets with the legal guardian, caregiver, parents, or parent and assesses how well equipped each family member is to provide support. If multiple problems are recognized, they agree on which problem to focus on first. Then the student is brought into the meeting, and the problem is described in specific terms. A concrete, measurable goal is established. The goal should be one that can be reached in a short amount of time (e.g., having 3 days of no fighting, completing homework, arriving to class on time). Positive and negative consequences are identified. The plan is put into writing. A monitoring system that the student agrees to is created. The plan is reviewed periodically. The family is given feedback (e.g., using a daily student rating card).

Comprehensive Social Contract

In this approach, all parties claim ownership for the student's problem (SLP, student, parent, administration, school personnel). Specific tasks are outlined for each person to carry out to ensure a positive change in the student's behavior. Realistic goals are set. An ongoing communication system is established. All parties agree to work together.

Cognitive Behavior Modification

Cognitive behavior modification is a metacognitive approach that requires the student to engage in self-reflection and self-awareness in a problem-solving fashion. Camp, Blom, Herbert, and Van Doornick (1977) created the "Think Aloud" method, which requires the student to answer four questions: (1) What is my problem? (2) What is my plan to solve the problem? (3) Am I using my plan? (4) How did I do?

Meichenbaum (2003) created a similar problem-solving approach using a five-step process: (a) What am I supposed to do? (b) I need to look at all possibilities. (c) I have to focus in and concentrate. (d) I have to make a choice. (e) How well did I do?

Role Reversal

In role reversal, the SLP and the student switch roles for a short time. The SLP recreates the conflict pretending to be the student. Then the student and the SLP enter into a positive student confrontation activity while continuing to remain in role reversal. Once an agreement has been reached, the SLP and the student honor it in their real roles.

Videotape

Videotaping is used most effectively with students who have cognitive disabilities. The SLP obtains permission from the parent or legal guardian to videotape the student. Then the SLP provides clear expectations and videotapes the student's compliant behaviors during a short session. The SLP sends the videotape home along with a list of specific, positive verbal praise comments that parents or caregivers could say to the student while they watch the videotape together. The student's family gets together and views the videotape with the student, who is the "movie star." Each member of the family offers positive praise statements as the videotape plays. The family congratulates the student on his or her pleasing behaviors and expresses the wish to view another tape of such behaviors in the future.

Audiotape

Audiotaping has been proved to be effective with students who use foul language in the classroom. The SLP obtains permission from the parent or legal guardian to audiotape the student. Then the SLP turns on the audiotape each day and lets the student know that if any foul language is heard, the tape will be replayed at the next parent-teacher conference. Another, more positive approach is to chart how many days in a row the audio tape did not contain any offensive language. The students are commended for their progress and told that the chart will be shown to parents at the next conference.

Using Older Students as Resources

High school students who have been disruptive can be recruited to work with younger students who are exhibiting disruptive behaviors. An hour once a week is sufficient. The high school student may participate during a study hall or be released an hour early from his or her academic program in order to participate. With parental permission, the SLP provides a brief overview of the younger student's disability, behavioral issues, and intervention plan. The older student is praised for being someone who has been given a special privilege to help another student. This type of social skills development may be written into IEPs for both the older student and the younger student.

Physical Considerations

The SLP must consider possible health considerations when a student exhibits radical behaviors. Students with communication disorders may not be capable of verbally describing what they are experiencing physically. They lack the ability to engage in **assertive communication**. The following vignette, from my own professional observation, highlights the possibility of a physical cause for behavior problems:

Tanisha suddenly jumped up from her seventh-hour science desk and started pacing back and forth in the back of the classroom. She clenched her fists and shook them in little circles in the air. After Tanisha ignored several directives from the teacher, she was kicked out of class and was sitting in a detention hall for the third time that week. By Monday of the following week, Tanisha's IEP team had convened a meeting to discuss adding behavior management goals to Tanisha's IEP. Tanisha was a 19-year-old high school student and her own legal guardian. The other members of the IEP team present at the meeting included Tanisha's foster home care worker, the transition coordinator, the SLP, Tanisha's job coach, her science teacher, the school psychologist, a teacher certified in the area of cognitive disabilities, and the director of special education.

The SLP was sitting next to Tanisha and noticed that Tanisha kept scratching her torso and rocking back and forth. Tanisha typically spoke in three-word phrases using a fast rate and slurred coarticulation. When the school psychologist asked Tanisha why she kept getting out of her seat and disrupting her classes, Tanisha responded, "Ititchesititchesititches." The school psychologist dismissed this as a nonsense utterance, but the SLP said, "I think Tanisha is telling us that something itches. Maybe she should be seen by the school nurse." Tanisha's foster home care worker confirmed that Tanisha had been scratching her torso for the past two weeks, ever since her return from visiting relatives during the winter break. The foster home care worker turned to Tanisha and asked, "Tanisha, do you itch?" Tanisha responded tearfully, "Yes! Ititchesititches ititches!" The IEP team decided not to add behavior management goals to Tanisha's IEP until the school nurse had a chance to examine Tanisha.

The next morning the school nurse confirmed the team's suspicions when she announced, "This looks like scabies." The school nurse phoned Tanisha's foster care worker; by the end of that day, Tanisha had been seen by a doctor at the local urgent care center. She did indeed have scabies. After proper treatment, Tanisha's classroom behaviors were again developmentally appropriate. No behavior management goals were added to her IEP.

This vignette demonstrates how important it is for the SLP to know the common manifestations of communicable diseases that are likely to affect children of school age. Lowe (1993) provided a brief overview of the signs and symptoms of common communicable childhood diseases, which are summarized in Table 6–1.

Table 6–1. Common Communicable Diseases Among School-Aged Children

Communicable Disease	Description
Scabies	A skin disease caused by the itch mite, which burrows under the skin, leaving a telltale grayish-white thin line. A raised rash characterized by pus-containing lesions, hives, and blisters may be present. Itching usually is intense and is worse at night.
Head lice (pediciulosis capitis)	An infestation that is highly contagious and easily transmitted through close contact close contact and sharing of brushes, combs, and hats. Lice cause intense itching of the scalp, and the resultant scratching often leads to superficial infections. Lice can transmit such diseases as typhus, trench fever, and relapsing fever.
Ringworm (tinea)	One of the most common superficial fungal infections. It can be transmitted from one person to another but more often is transmitted from an infected animal to a person. Ringworm of the scalp often is seen in school children. The hair loses its pigmentation, and small crusting pustules are seen at the base of the hair follicle; red scales develop later. The hair falls out, giving rise to the characteristic bald patches.
Pinkeye (conjunctivitis)	An inflammation of the eye caused by an infectious organism that may be bacterial or viral, or by irritants such as dust or sand, or may be allergy related. Itching, redness, swelling, tearing of the eye, and sensitivity to light are common clinical manifestations.
Pinworm infestations (enterobiasis)	A common childhood malady. The worms live in the rectum or colon but emerge onto the skin around the anus at night, where they lay their eggs and cause intense itching. In females, the worms may spread to the vaginal area, causing intense itching.

continues

Table 6–1. *continued*

Communicable Disease	Description
Whooping cough (pertussis)	A bacterial respiratory infection. It is transmitted by droplets sprayed from the mouth during talking or coughing or by direct contact with articles contaminated by the organism. Whooping cough usually begins with a fever, runny nose, sneezing, and coughing. After about 2 weeks, the cough becomes spasmodic. Severe respiratory complications may ensue.
Chickenpox (varicella)	An acute communicable disease caused by a virus. Fever, headache, nausea, and vomiting generally precede a rash consisting of crops of lesions on the neck or trunk, which soon spread to the face, scalp, mucous membranes, and extremities. The lesions first appear as small, flat red blotches. Later these become raised vesicles that are found to contain pus in 2 to 4 days. Reye's syndrome, encephalitis, and meningitis may occur after an outbreak of chickenpox.
German measles (rubella)	A viral infection that causes mild illness in children. A blotchy rash that appears first on the face and then spreads to the trunk and extremities is common. Pinpoint rose-red spots also may be seen on the soft palate. The affected child exhibits fatigue, lack of appetite, slight temperature elevation, and swollen glands. Most children are routinely immunized by about 15 months of age with the combined measles-mumps-rubella (MMR) vaccine. Because additional outbreaks are possible, a second immunization when the child enters middle school is recommended. The child with rubella must be isolated to prevent exposure to pregnant women and possible subsequent damage to their unborn children.
Measles (rubeola)	An acute illness caused by a virus. The disease generally begins with an upper respiratory tract infection; the affected child has a high fever, cough, sore throat, red and teary eyes that are sensitive to light, and possibly swollen glands. Spots with grayish centers surrounded by red irregular rings appear in the mouth. A red blotchy rash appears 4 to 5 days after the initial signs. Sometimes the brain, heart, and other organs may be permanently damaged. Pneumonia and obstructive laryngitis and tracheitis are respiratory tract complications that also may follow.
Mumps (parotitis)	A disease of viral origin that affects the parotid glands. A child with this infection experiences headache, muscle aches, pain behind the ear(s) with chewing or swallowing, and fever. A severe complication of mumps is encephalitis.
Acquired immunodeficiency syndrome (AIDS)	A fatal disease of the immune system that leaves the body without adequate protection against disease-producing organisms. Seventy-seven percent of infected children acquired the disease after birth from infected mothers.
Reye's syndrome	An acute disorder that affects many body systems, especially the liver and brain. It occurs most often after a viral infection such as influenza or chickenpox. Administration of aspirin has been associated with development of this syndrome. Lethargy, drowsiness, nausea, vomiting, irritability, and general lack of interest are common.
Lyme disease	A disease caused by a small spiral-shaped bacterium that is transmitted to humans primarily by the bite of the small deer tick, bear tick, or dog tick. A skin lesion begins as a small, round, raised reddened area at the site of the bite. It soon spreads to several inches in diameter (the "target" lesion). The lymph glands become tender, and the child may complain of fatigue, headache, fever, body ache, and chills.
Mononucleosis (Epstein-Barr virus infection)	A viral infection that is transmitted through saliva. Signs and symptoms include weakness, fatigue, sore throat, fever, swollen lymph nodes and tonsils, headache, skin rash, loss of appetite, and night sweats.

Sources: Lowe (1993), NCIDC-CDC (2007).

The school-based SLP also must be aware of the effects of lead poisoning. The following vignette, from a case from the personal records of Gwen Robl, a highly experienced SLP, is presented as a concrete example:

Two brothers, both in sixth grade (because the older one had been retained) moved into our district last fall. One had a history of special education and the other did not. Records were very difficult to track down because the family had moved several times. I met both boys and was concerned about their needs and that their language characteristics were not just delayed, they were disordered. To make a long story short, I talked with the social worker who was going to conduct a parent interview and obtain case histories. I emphasized the need to acquire detailed information about the boys' developmental histories. It was discovered that both boys had high blood levels of lead during very early developmental years. Lead poisoning can result in learning disabilities, language disabilities, AD/HD, and so on.

These boys probably demonstrated the largest discrepancies between visual hands-on versus verbal learning characteristics that I had seen in my 30-plus years of professional work. Both boys confused words receptively and expressively that were phonetically similar, such as pitch/pinch or riddle/rhythm. They both demonstrated memory deficits, attention deficits, and limited verbal expression.

The younger boy received special education for behavioral concerns. Considering that his visual IQ exceeded 120, his verbal IQ was 100, and his verbal language IQ was in the low 80s with verbal facility—1.75 standard deviations below the mean on all measures, it's no wonder he showed signs of depression and withdrawal. He spoke exceedingly slowly and included every detail; he did not summarize or give main ideas. His peers would either prod him to get to the point or stop listening before he finished expressing his thoughts. He knew he had a good idea but could not get anyone to listen to him. This caused him extreme frustration; he often became angry, and aggressive. This was one of the few

students that I provided services for as a related service. (G. Robl, personal communication, July 18, 2005)

Effective Conflict Resolution Strategies to Use with Adults

The school-based SLP also must know ways to diffuse conflict between adults. Human beings have many different ways of resolving conflict because human beings have many different personality types. A competitive person may view the conflict as a win-lose situation, whereas a passive person may opt to avoid or accommodate as the preferred solution. Collaboration and compromise are not easily achieved. The SLP is wise to engage in self-reflection, to understand his or her own personality type, and to seek specific training in effective conflict resolution. Webne-Behrman (2005) offered eight steps for effective conflict resolution, summarized next.

Step 1

"Know thyself"—and take care of yourself. Learn what your own biases are. Learn what makes you angry and why. Analyze how you handled conflict in the past and consider what alternatives would have yielded a more positive outcome. Eating healthy foods, getting ample sleep, and exercising may make it easier to cope with stress. Confiding in a trusted friend or coworker also may prove useful.

Step 2

Clarify personal needs threatened by the dispute. Webne-Behrman identified three types of needs that must be addressed: *substantive needs* (i.e., knowing the problem that needs to be solved); *procedural needs* (i.e., knowing specific strategies and how to use them effectively); and *psychological needs* (i.e., knowing how to establish a safe environment that allows all parties to be honest and open in their communications). All three types of needs must be addressed in any conflict. Thinking about the negative outcomes if the conflict is not resolved helps clarify the three types of needs. Webne-Behrman encourages reflection and identification of the *best* alternative to a negotiated agreement (**BATNA**), the *worst* alternative to a negotiated agreement (**WATNA**), and the *most likely* alternative to a negotiated agreement (**MLATNA**). By thinking through these alternatives, it is possible to identify the best solution and why it is better than other alternatives as a way to meet one's needs. The focus should be limited to only two or three priority issues: What are the needs that are most threatened and most important to be negotiated? How do they relate to the other person's situation?

Webne-Behman (2005) offers "ground rules" to apply in conflict resolution. His work is summarized here:

- One person will speak at a time.
- We shall listen to one another with respect.
- We shall seek to understand one another's point of view, and to be flexible about differing perceptions of the issues at hand.
- We shall agree to honor the confidentiality of our discussions.

Step 3

The location and time of the negotiations must be carefully selected. The space should be neutral and not owned by one party or the other. The space should allow privacy, and the furniture should allow for face-to-face conversation. A round table is better than a rectangular one. The chairs should be the same height so that each participant feels like an equal. The time is of the meeting is just as important as the location. If time is limited, the first meeting may be devoted to just identifying the problem. Another meeting should be set up for more in-depth dialogue, with ample time for the discussion. Facilitators, mediators, and advocates may attend subsequent meetings.

Step 4

Use active listening skills. Sometimes it is necessary to go through an anger management program before it is possible to achieve this outcome. When a person is in control of emotions and able to listen to another's perspective, additional information may be gained that actually helps meet that person's needs.

Step 5

Communicate your own concerns in a way that makes it likely for them to be heard and understood by the other person. Use "I messages" as a tool for clarification. Be prepared to deal with hostility. The same event may trigger very different perceptions in two different people. Both parties must define the problem in similar terms. Differing priorities must be identified.

Step 6

Be flexible if the focus of the negotiation needs to shift. Brainstorm regarding all possible solutions without judgment. Then identify and define the criteria by which each idea is judged. Summarize solutions in writing and restate them to provide assurance that all parties actually agree on the solution.

Step 7

Manage impasse with calm and respect. Clarify feelings; stay focused on the needs; and take structured breaks. It is unlikely that a solution will result when emotions escalate. A structured break allows all parties to maintain the focus, renew energy, and keep their emotions in check. It also gives each party a chance to reflect on his or her MLANTA and to weigh it against the BATNA and the WATNA. Such reflections may show that continued negotiations are important so that needs may still be met. If a third party mediator or facilitator is involved, breaks allow opportunities for caucus. When impasse occurs, verbalize the feelings that the impasse is creating. Sometimes it is helpful to reframe the issue or change the focus from a substantive need to a procedural need or psychological need. Breaking the issue into manageable parts is another useful strategy. Restating the problem and assuring the other party that his or her point of view is understood constitute a strategy that may help overcome the impasse. Flexibility in thinking is important. Identify the elements that are mutually acceptable. Reaffirm the ground rules.

Step 8

Finally, build an agreement that works. It is likely that all parties will feel exhaustion, rather than excitement, when an agreement has been achieved. In a compromise situation, neither party is overjoyed by the solution, but both are willing to accept it. After all of the hard work that they invested, both parties may feel disheartened over the actual solution but recognize it as a necessary plan to move forward. Identify areas of agreement in writing. Then take time to reflect and review. Decide whether the agreement is actually fair, balanced, and realistic. Is there a way to implement the agreement? Make sure that all parties involved understand their roles and responsibilities. Build in an accountability system to ensured that each party will actually follow through on assigned responsibilities. Make a plan to address future problems, should they arise. Communicate with each other about possible roadblocks to the implementation of the solution. Evaluate the progress of the solution and develop a communication avenue.

Summary

Behavioral issues, conflict resolution, and problem solving go with the territory of public school services. Graduate programs and postgraduate inservices that focus on remediation approaches are not enough. The SLP also must learn (1) positive, proactive strategies to help students learn how to communicate in the most effective ways; (2) how

to create a proactive plan that includes rules, rewards, and consequences; (3) how to teach that plan to students and communicate that plan to colleagues, administrators, and parents or caregivers; (4) how to be consistent and focus on positive growth for each student; (5) how to acknowledge the students' feelings even when he or she must provide a consequence for the students' actions; (6) how to consider child and adolescent development; (7) how to create a safe environment and build a community culture; (8) how to consider the physical needs of the students; (9) how to collaborate with others; (10) how to teach metacognitive exercises to promote self-reflection in students as they develop problem-solving skills; (11) how to use conflict resolution strategies; and (12) how to implement conflict resolution strategies in the school setting.

Questions for Application and Review

1. List some of the reasons that students today exhibit behaviors that require modification.
2. Change the following phrases to "do" statements from "don't" statements: *don't run*; *don't yell*; *don't talk out of turn*; *don't hit*; *don't leave the classroom without a pass*.
3. Give one example of when foreshadowing expectations with high school students would be appropriate.
4. Give one example of when it would be essential to know basic child development when working with a middle school student.
5. List three ways to create a safe environment.
6. Why is it important to consider the physical needs of the student?
7. How can burnout be prevented among educators dealing with students who have severe behavioral issues?
8. Why is it important to teach metacognitive and self-reflective strategies to students?
9. What is meant by the term *community culture*?
10. What are the eight steps of conflict resolution strategies recommended by Webne-Behrman (2005)?

References

Brinton, B., Fujiki, M., & Higbee, L. (1998). Participation in cooperative learning activities by children with specific language impairment. *Journal of Speech, Language, and Hearing Research, 41,* 1193-1206.

Canter, L., & Canter, M. (1985). *Assertive discipline.* Santa Monica, CA: Canter Associates.

Camp, B., Blom, G., Herbert, F., & Van Doornick, W. (1977). Think aloud: A program for developing self-control in young aggressive boys. *Journal of Abnormal Child Psychology, 5,* 157-169.

Carr, E. G., Levin, L., McConnachie, G., Carlson, J. I., Kemp, D. C, & Smith, C. E. (1994). *Communication-based intervention for problem behaviors.* Baltimore: Brookes.

Children's Defense Fund. (2005). *A moral outrage: One American child or teen killed by gunfire nearly every 3 hours.* Retrieved January 31, 2005, from http://www.childrensdefense.org/site/PageServer?pagename=pressreleases_default

Curwin, R., & Mendler, A. (1999). *Discipline with dignity.* Alexandria, VA: Association for Supervision and Curriculum Development.

Fujiki, M., Brinton, B., & Clarke, D. (2002). Emotion regulation in children with specific language impairment. *Language, Speech, and Hearing Services in Schools, 33,* 102-111.

Fukiki, M. Brinton, B., Hart, C. H., & Fitzgerald, A. H. (1999). Peer acceptance and friendship in children with specific language impairment. *Topics in Language Disorders, 1992,* 49-69.

Fujiki, M., Brinton, B., Isaacson, T., & summers, C. (2001). Social behaviors of children with language impairment on the playground. *Language, Speech, and Hearing Services in Schools, 32,* 101-113.

Fujiki, M. Spackman, M.P., Brinton, B., & Hall, A. (2004). The relationship of language and emotion regulation skills to reticence in children with specific language impairment. *Journal of Speech, Language, and Hearing Research, 47,* 637-646.

Hegde, M. N., & Davis, D. (1995). *Clinical methods and practicum in speech-language pathology* (2nd ed.). San Diego, CA: Singular.

Johnson, D. W., & Johnson, R. T. (1995). *Reducing school violence through conflict resolution.* Alexandria, VA: Association for Supervision and Curriculum Development.

Johnston, S. S., & Reichle, J. (1993). Designing and implementing interventions to decrease challenging behavior. *Language, Speech, and Hearing Services in Schools, 24,* 225-235.

Kohn, A. (1996). *Beyond discipline from compliance to community.* Alexandria, VA: Association for Supervision and Curriculum Development.

Lowe, R. J. (1993). *Speech-language pathology & related professions in the schools.* Needham Heights, MA: Allyn & Bacon.

Meichenbaum, D. (2003). *Treatment of individuals with anger control problems and aggressive behavior.* Clearwater, FL: Institute Press.

National Center for Infectious Diseases Centers for Disease control and Prevention (2007). Epstein-Barr virus and infectious monomucleosis. Retrieved December 15, 2007 from, http://www.cdc.gov/ncidod/diseases/ebv.htm

Nungesser, N. R., & Watkins, R. V. (2005). Preschool teachers' perceptions and reactions to challenging classroom behavior: Implications for speech-language pathologists. *Language, Speech, and Hearing Services in Schools, 36,* 139-151.

Olson, J. (2007). What about behavior? Considerations for speech-language pathologists. Retrieved August 28, 2007, from http://www.speechpathology.com

Redmond, S. M., & Rice, J. L. (1998). The socioemotional behaviors of children with SLI: Social adaptation or social deviance? *Journal of Speech, Language, and Hearing Research, 41,* 688-700.

Warner, J., & Bryan, C. (1995). *The unauthorized teacher's survival guide.* Indianapolis, IN: Park Avenue.

Webne-Behrman, H. (2005). *Eight steps for conflict resolution.* Retrieved January 20, 2005, from http://www.ohrd.wisc.edu/onlinetraining/resolution/index.asp

White, P. (2004). *Managing threatening confrontations.* Verona, WI: Attainment.

Chapter 7

CULTURAL COMPETENCE IN COMMUNICATION

RELATED VOCABULARY

accent   A set of stress and intonation patterns unique to a specific language.

authentic assessment   A method of assessment that requires students to perform, produce, or demonstrate skills representing realistic learning demands.

bias   A preference for the familiar and comfortable.

dialect   A variation in pronunciation, vocabulary, and idiomatic use of language that is specific to a geographical region.

discrimination   Distinguishing one thing from among others; a distinction and favor of what is comfortable and familiar.

dynamic assessment   A method of conducting assessment that is interactive. The examiner observes the result of modifying instructional input on the learning process and discovers what works best to maximize an individual's learning.

ethnocentrism   A belief that one's own culture and beliefs are superior to those of others.

fast-mapping   The process by which people rapidly learn novel words on brief but intense exposure.

interpersonal communication   Communication between two or more people.

paralanguage silence The amount of time between when one person finishes speaking and another begins speaking that is socially accepted within a culture.

prejudice A judgment that is based on emotion or some other irrational factor, rather than on the relevant facts.

projected cognitive similarity The assumption that one knows how another is thinking based on one's own perceptions.

prototype A mental representation based on general characteristics that are not fixed or rigid. A prototype is fluid and dynamic and open to new definitions.

stereotype A mental representation based on specific characteristics that are rigid.

Introduction

According to the U.S. Census of 2000, 18.4% of children 5 to 17 years of age speak a language other than English. The proportion of children from Latino cultures is the fastest growing, accounting for 16.3% of children enrolled in public elementary and secondary schools. In 2000, the school-age population also was composed of 61.2% white, 17.2% black, 4.1% Asian or Pacific Islander, and 1.2% American Indian/Alaskan Native (U.S. Census Bureau, 2000). Unquestionably, the school-age population across the United States is rich in diversity. Thus, school-based speech-language pathologists (SLPs) are ethically bound to become culturally competent and also to be able to distinguish a communication delay or disorder from a communication difference, particularly in the realm of language. The American Speech-Language-Hearing Association (ASHA) Code of Ethics (ASHA, 2003) proclaimed: "Individuals shall honor their responsibility to hold paramount the welfare of persons they serve professionally" (p. 2), and "Individuals shall not discriminate in the delivery of professional services on the basis of race or ethnicity, gender, age, religion, national origin, sexual orientation, or disability" (p. 5).

Cultural competency begins with an understanding of one's own experiences. Communication is at the heart of one's own experience. Cheng (1999a) has eloquently made this point: "The most precious thing that human beings possess is the ability to use language to communicate. People use languages in various forms and speak them in different ways to express what they think they mean. Human communication is diverse and unpredictable" (p. vi.). As noted by Varner and Beamer (1995), most people think that their culture is the best way of life and that persons from other cultures should try to adopt or imitate their culture. Hall (1976) reminds us that the roads to truth are many and that no culture is better equipped than others to search for it. Hofstede (1991) recommended that the first step in surviving in a multicultural world is to understand that people do not need to think, feel, or act in the same way in order to agree or cooperate. Varner and Beamer (1995) explained that people can agree to be different, celebrate their own culture, and celebrate other cultures because they are different; the more is known about other cultures, the more about one's own culture will become evident. This knowledge of one's own culture makes it easier to embark on a metacognitive journey, examine the assumptions and attitudes one has acquired, and learn to appreciate the cultures of others.

Varner and Beamer described some typical *reactions to unfamiliar cultures*. Their work in this area can be summarized as follows:

- Assumption of superiority. When confronted with a cultural difference, most people respond by thinking their way is the better way. The SLP must be aware of this typical reaction when assessing and evaluating the needs of a student from a different culture.

- **Ethnocentrism**. Members of other cultures are convinced, deep down in their heart of hearts, that their own culture is the "right" one. People everywhere tend to assume that their own culture is the norm, and to assess all other cultures by how closely they resemble their own. Most people, especially those with little experience of other cultures, believe that their own culture (ethnicity) is at the center of human experience.

- Assumption of universality. Culture is a whole view of the universe from which people assess the meaning of life and their appropriate response to it. The assumption that one knows how another is thinking, based on how one sees things, is called **projected cognitive similarity**. It occurs when someone else's perceptions, judgments, attitudes, and values are assumed to be like one's own. This can lead to disrupted communication and even conflict.

- Mental representations. All people use executive functions to organize and make sense of their world. It is important to be aware of the difference between **stereotype** and **prototype**. The term *stereotype* came from the days of the printing press, when type set in one frame was identically reproduced in another frame. A stereotype is fixed and rigid. By contrast, a *prototype* is a mental representation based on general charac-

teristics that are not fixed or rigid. A prototype is fluid and dynamic and open to new definitions.

- **Bias**. A bias is a preference for the familiar and comfortable.

- **Discrimination**. When biases are acted on, the actor is showing discrimination or **prejudice.** Discrimination is the act of sifting out and selecting according to bias toward something or someone.

- **Prejudice**. Prejudice is a judgment that is based on emotion or some other irrational factor, but not on the relevant facts. Prejudice exists *in spite of* the facts. A prejudice usually is negative, and because it is not grounded in fact, it can be called an irrational bias. Prejudice often is accompanied by or based on suspicion, fear, hate, or contempt.

Battle (1998) offered seven points of wisdom for SLPs embarking on the journey to become culturally competent. First, it is important to learn and use the name for a culture that is preferred by its own members. A person from Colombia prefers to be referred to as *Colombian*, not *Hispanic*. Second, generic terms or descriptions of race should not be used to refer to a culture, and the term *minority* should be avoided in this context. In many areas of the country, what is commonly referred to as a minority group may actually constitute more than 50% of the population. Thus, the designation *minority* cannot be assumed to be correct. Third, it should not be assumed that all African Americans speak African American English, for example, or that all white persons speak Standard American English. It is even possible for African American English to be the preferred **dialect** (as opposed to **accent**) of a white child. Fourth, it is important to avoid terms that have negative connotations, such as *culturally deprived* or *at-risk minority*. Poverty cuts across all cultural groups. Fifth, the SLP should become aware of and avoid using color-symbolic or ethnoculturally specific language that supports stereotypes (e.g., "black sheep," "white lie," "Indian giver," "Chinese fire drill"). Sixth, the SLP also should become knowledgeable about the nonverbal aspects of a culture (e.g., greeting style, distance between speakers, eye contact, touch). Finally, the SLP should develop a culture-specific sense of the importance of an individual in relation to the group and how this role may vary among different cultures.

Interview and Case History

School-based SLPs must consider cultural diversity at every step of the individualized education program (IEP) process and with every aspect of assessment, intervention, consultation, and collaboration. The SLP must be aware of culture differences when seeking case history information. Harris (1993) cautioned that establishing rapport can be heavily influenced by the type of topics addressed, questions asked, and the manner in which each question is asked. Questions typically asked during a case history (regarding birth history, place of residence, the nature of the client's communication difficulties, and so on) may be considered by some clients as being too personal, intrusive, inappropriate, or irrelevant. In some Native American communities, for example, the mere mention or discussion of an individual's disability can be viewed as potentially putting that person at risk for greater difficulties. For some clients, questions as simple as "Where do you live?" can be viewed with suspicion. Clients who have a high level of cultural mistrust, as defined by Terrell and Terrell (1996), may misinterpret this type of question as an indirect attempt to obtain private information, such as the client's socioeconomic or immigration status (i.e., illegal versus legal). Either of these can have a negative impact on the amount of information that clients are willing to disclose.

Battle (1998) recommended asking someone who knows the client's cultural community to review case history questions before the interview to determine their cultural appropriateness. The cultural mentor may be an elderly person, an extended family member, a religious leader, another educator, a physician, a social worker, or a local political leader. By enlisting the assistance of a cultural mentor, the SLP may gain important knowledge about the family's views on spirituality, holidays, history, traditions, education, art, music, family structure, the role of women, sleeping patterns, food preferences, feeding patterns, standards for hygiene, toilet training, affective attitudes, behavioral expectations, work ethic, health care, time orientation, eye contact, **paralanguage silence**, personal space and proximity, facial expressions, head nodding, voice loudness, voice inflection and stress, social rituals, use of names, use of humor and sarcasm, patterns within conversational turn taking, phonological and linguistic differences, attitudes toward pets and animals, and beliefs related to disabilities. These are just a few of the cultural, social interaction, and communication features that may influence how successful the SLP will be in obtaining case history information.

The SLP and other team members must be respectful of the family's culture when collaborating during the IEP process. Something as simple as providing tea, rather than coffee, during a conference meeting may make a big difference in how comfortable the family members may feel during the meeting. Interaction style also is an important consideration. Table 7–1 depicts some differences between African-American cultures and other cultures with respect to interaction styles.

Assessment Tools

The SLP must consider cultural diversity when selecting standardized assessment tools (ASHA, 2004; Crowley, 2003; Taylor, 1986; Wolfram, 1976). Although this sounds relatively simple, determining the norms and expectations of a student's speech community can in fact be quite challenging. For instance, a student may come from a speech community where Hmong is spoken. In school, the student is exposed primarily to Standard American English. In the home community, the student is exposed to several dialects of Hmong and several dialects of English (including Spanish-Influenced English and African American English). Among his friends in the community, he usually "code switches" between Hmong, Spanish-Influenced

Table 7–1. Interaction Styles of African Americans Contrasted with Other Cultural Groups

Interaction Feature	African-American Culture	Opposing View
Touching	Another person touching one's hair is offensive	Another person touching one's hair is a sign of affection
Eye contact	Indirect eye contact during speaking is a sign of attentiveness and respect	Direct eye contact during listening and indirect eye contact during speaking are signs of attention and respect
Public behavior	Public behavior may be emotionally intense, dynamic, and demonstrative	Public behavior is modest and emotionally restrained; emotional displays are seen as irresponsible or in bad taste
Conflict	A clear distinction exists between argument and fight; verbal sparring is not necessarily a precursor to violence	Heated arguments suggest that violence is imminent
Sharing personal information	Asking personal questions of someone a person has met for the first time is seen as improper and intrusive	Inquiring about jobs, family, and so forth of someone a person has met for the first time is seen as friendly
Reaction to direct questions	The use of direct questions is sometimes seen as harassment	The use of direct questions for personal information is permissible
Turn taking in conversation	Interruption during conversation usually is tolerated; access to speaking is granted to the person who is most assertive	Rules of turn taking in conversation dictate that one person speaks at a time until all of that person's points are made
Conversational additions	Conversations are regarded as private between the recognized participants	Adding a point of information or insight to a conversation in which a person is not engaged is seen as being helpful
Interpretation of silence	Silence denotes refutation of accusation	Silence denotes acceptance of an accusation

Sources: Freiberg, 1997; Taylor, 1986.

English, African American English, and Standard American English. What, then, is that student's speech community, and what standard should be applied? Zentella (1997) documented that in New York City, SLPs frequently are asked to evaluate students from bilingual or multidialectal homes and communities in which several dialects of Spanish and English are spoken. The children from these communities receive a variety of linguistic inputs, such as Standard Spanish, Standard Puerto Rican Spanish, Standard Dominican Spanish, Vernacular Spanish, Standard English, Puerto Rican English,

Hispanized English, and African American English. Speakers from these communities often switch between dialects of one language or between dialects of the two different languages, depending on the person to whom they are speaking, where they are speaking, what they are speaking about, and why they are speaking.

School-based SLPs have been frustrated by the lack of appropriate assessment tools available for use with today's diverse school-age populations. As discussed by Crowley and Valenti (2004), biases in assessment tools include more than the form of the language. Biases also include the manner in which language is used. Communication is determined by cultural factors. Most testing procedures do not take the cultural aspects of communication into consideration. Heath (1982) pointed out that the cultural norm of labeling objects and pictures in books by parents of mainstream American middle class is not part of parenting styles among other cultures. Yet standardized tests often require the child to sit, look at pictures, and label objects during assessment of vocabulary development. As documented by Pena and Quinn (1997), labeling objects and pictures in books is not part of certain Puerto Rican and African-American cultures.

School-based SLPs must be concerned about discrimination at all age levels, especially at the preschool level, when adult-child interactions are particularly tender. Schraeder, Quinn, Stockman, and Miller (1999) pointed out three major concerns. First, few tests include persons from low-income families in the normative populations, regardless of race. Second, the interaction style demanded by many standardized tests does not match the interaction style of preschool children. Crago (1992) documented that preschool children typically engage in parallel, rather than interactive, play. Adler (1993) and Schieffelin (1994) also documented that children from different cultures relate differently during adult-child interactions. Third, the definition of what constitutes a communication delay or disorder has broadened over the past two decades. Standardized tests often focus exclusively on phonology, syntax, comprehension, and auditory processing skills. As documented by Crais (1994, 1995), McCauley and Swisher (1984), McFadden (1996), and Wetherby and Prizant (1992), other aspects of communication, such as the interaction style of the conversational partner, discourse parameters, materials used, the setting, the task, and the demands on information processing, also are important aspects to assess.

Informal assessment tools also have proved to be problematic. Crowley and Valenti (2004) and Heath (1982) documented that cultural biases are present in alternative assessment procedures. For example, the quality and quantity of a language sample that is collected may be significantly affected by social and cultural factors. For example, a child

of any culture may be reticent in speaking with an unfamiliar adult about something uninteresting in an unfamiliar setting; however, the child's linguistic performance may be judged substandard by an educator with unconscious bias toward the child's cultural group. Moreover, if the elicitation task is culturally unfamiliar to the student, the language sample may not yield true production abilities, as in a language sample that is collected through a story-retell task. This elicitation task can be biased if the child has not had experience telling or hearing stories because it is not part of his or her culture to do so.

When a language sample is being collected for analysis, Adler (1993) and Hegde and Davis (1995) recommended acquiring more than one sample in different settings and with different people. In this way the SLP is able to analyze not only the various parameters of language, articulation, voice, fluency, and pragmatics but also which antecedents enhance linguistic performance, diminish performance, or appear to have no impact. Collecting language samples while the student is interacting with various family members also may give the SLP insight into which family member seems the most appropriate candidate for working with the student in a home carryover program.

When conducting a classroom observation, the SLP must be aware of the differences between the expectations of the American classroom and the expectations of parents from various cultural and ethnic groups. Table 7–2 illustrates the contrast between American and Asian cultures in terms of expectations of classroom behaviors.

The SLP must be aware of the influences of culture on the student's learning style. Freiberg (1997) cautioned that communication characteristics and the learning styles that are typical in Native American Indian cultures may be misinterpreted as characteristics that warrant a referral for special education. Such characteristics include the following:

■ Reliance on nonverbal communication. A nod, smile, or shrug, for example, may be used for this purpose.
■ Saying only what is necessary. A student may answer simply "yes" or "no," for

Table 7–2. Comparison of American and Asian Cultures for Expectations of Classroom Behaviors

Behavioral Feature	Expectations of American Classroom Teacher	Expectations of Parents from an Asian Culture
Student participation	Students need to actively participate in classroom activities and discussions	Students are to be quiet and obedient
Student initiative	Students need to be creative	Students should be told what to do and what not to do
Mode of learning	Students learn through inquiries and debate	Students learn through memorization and observation
Student-teacher interaction	Asian students do well on their own	Teachers need to teach; students need to study
Level of thinking	Critical thinking and analytical thinking are important	Factual information is important
Problem solving	Creativity and fantasy are encouraged	Students should be taught the steps to solve problems
Question asking	Students need to ask questions	Teachers are not to be challenged

Sources: Cheng, 1991; Freiberg, 1997.

example, or fail to elaborate when to do so is expected.

- Speaking in a soft, low-pitched voice. In these cultures, loud, projected speech is to be avoided in conversation because it indicates aggression or anger.
- Displaying a deep sense of humor and an ability to see humor in life. Educators may perceive such behavior as rude or as a manifestation of emotional imbalance.
- Long pauses in conversation. A student who is deliberate in giving a response, rather than providing instant answers, may be perceived by educators as not knowing the answer or as having an expressive language or auditory processing problem.

A majority of middle class white students begin school as auditory learners. They have been bombarded with verbal information since early childhood. Their parents talk to them a great deal. They are encouraged to talk, to learn new words, and to express their ideas. Their parents have taught them many things through verbal explanations. By contrast, many Native American Indian students are visual learners. They have learned to do things by observing. When their parents instruct them in new skills, they do so mostly by showing them how to do something. The students learn to do the things their parents do by imitating them. They have been taught that children should not be talking continuously. These children have done most of their learning through direct experience and participation in real-world activities.

The issue becomes even more complex when the SLP considers factors related to code switching and code mixing. Major differences exist between discourse rules in different cultures. Cheng (1999b) reported results from a study conducted by Bishop (1988), who observed Vietnamese children living in America. The children were using English discourse rules along with those of their home culture, simultaneously engaging two different codes —one linguistic and one pragmatic. This study showed the importance of knowing not only the linguistic rules but also the cultural rules of a new language.

When assessing students who are English language learners, the SLP must be aware of deeper levels of language proficiency, as well as the surface levels of language proficiency. Cummins (1984) describes two levels of English proficiency:

1. Basic **interpersonal communication** skill (BICS)—required for social communication. BICS is the type of communication students acquire first because it is rich in the context of the situation and in social interaction. Cummins argues that students usually are able to acquire BICS within 2 years.
2. Cognitive academic language proficiency (CALP)—required for academic learning that is new and unfamiliar. Less information is derived from the immediate context. CALP requires students to learn exclusively from the language used to convey the message. They are not able to rely on situational cues. Cummins argues that CALP proficiency may take 5 to 7 years or longer to achieve.

The classroom teacher may wrongly refer an English language learner (ELL) who has acquired BICS for special education services. For example, the teacher may see an adolescent ELL joking in the halls with other students, obtaining a driver's license, and acquiring a part-time job. On the basis of such observations, the teacher believes that for all practical purposes, this student has well-developed functional English language skills. When that adolescent with BICS proficiency enters the classroom, however, he or she may struggle with academic performance if the student has not yet achieved CALP. Students need to acquire proficiencies along a continuum of BICS to CALP, and the SLP must know how to assess and evaluate those students' language proficiency with respect to academic performance, as well as social skills performance. Figure 7–1 shows four quadrants that illustrate the effect of context on cognitive demand.

Cummins also makes the point that students who have acquired BICS may be able to function proficiently at the lower levels of Bloom's (1956) taxonomy (i.e., knowledge, comprehension, and application), but not at the higher levels (i.e., analysis, synthesis, and evaluation), because of the advanced language complexity required to respond to academic tasks that address the higher levels of the taxonomy.

New Approaches to Assessment

It is not realistic for the school-based SLP to become proficient in every language that is spoken within the school-age population. A solution that shows promise is to assess the student's language-learning ability, rather than language proficiency. Two new approaches of measuring language-learning ability that are currently being researched are **fast-mapping** (also known as quick incidental learning) and **dynamic assessment.** Hwa-Froelich,

Context rich	**Context reduced**
Cognitively demanding	Cognitively demanding
Context rich	**Context reduced**
Cognitively undemanding	Cognitively undemanding

Figure 7–1. Effect of context on cognitive academic language proficiency.

Westby, and Schommer-Aikins (2000) described fast-mapping as when children participate in an activity in which they hear novel or unfamiliar words. The caregiver or educator does not attempt to teach the words but provides opportunities for the child to hear the words, morphemes, or concepts. Children are then presented with tasks requiring them to display their ability to comprehend and produce the novel or unfamiliar words. Dollaghan (1985), Rice, Buhr, and Nemeth (1990), and Oetting, Rice, and Swank (1995) demonstrated that children with language impairments exhibit a slower rate of language learnability than that observed in children who demonstrate typically developing language acquisition. Thus, fast-mapping shows promise as a way to assess a student's language-learning ability ("language learnability") without having to consider the child's native language. Hwa-Froelich (2000) and colleagues (Hwa-Froelich et al., 2000) indicated that dynamic assessment differs from fast-mapping in that the examiner actively teaches and carefully "mediates" the child's learning. A test-teach-test sequence is employed.

Another new approach being researched is **authentic assessment**. Udvari and Thousand (1995) defined authentic assessment as occurring when students are expected to perform, produce, or otherwise demonstrate skills that represent realistic learning demands. The contexts of the assessments are real-life settings in and out of the classroom without contrived and standardized conditions. Rosin and Gill (1997) and Schraeder and associates (1999) determined that authentic assessment differs from language sample analysis because it adds contextual, performance dimensions, and instructional linkages to the analysis of the child's communication competence.

The difference between BICS and CALP must be taken into consideration when an authentic assessment approach is used. Westby (2000) created the *Playscale* that reflected five possible play-language relationships. Three statements on the scale described typical cognitive and language development characteristics, and two statements described characteristics of disordered communication. A similar play-language scale that reflects the continuum of BICS to CALP could be developed as a useful authentic assessment tool.

Other alternatives to standardized assessment tools include criterion-referenced tools, client specific tools, dynamic assessment, and portfolio assessment. Criterion-referenced and dynamic assessments and client-specific and portfolio assessments are advantageous because the student need not be compared to students in a normative sample or population. These alternatives establish a set of characteristics, or rubrics, that the student is expected to achieve. In the case of dynamic assessment and client-specific assessment, the student's performance compared with his or her own baseline performance to determine the rate of progress. In the case of criterion-referenced and portfolio systems, the student is judged on how well he or she has met the defined criteria. Section VI of the *ASHA Directory of Speech-Language Pathology Assessment Instruments* offers a description of evaluation tools designed for use with culturally and linguistically diverse populations (ASHA, 2007). The ASHA Directory is available at www.asha.org/policy

Cultural Considerations Related to Intervention

The need for cultural competency does not end with collaboration, assessment, and evaluation. The SLP also must be aware of cultural differences when engaging in intervention. Burnette (1999) recommended *teaching behaviors* that may build a stronger teaching-learning relationship with culturally diverse students:

■ Appreciate and accommodate the similarities and differences among the students' cultures. Effective teachers of culturally diverse students enthusiastically acknowledge both individual and cultural differences and identify these differences in a positive manner. This positive identification creates a basis for developing effective communication and instructional strategies. Social skills such as respect and cross-cultural understanding can be modeled, taught, prompted, and reinforced by the teacher. Teachers should be introspective in recognizing their own possible biases and how they may affect overall teaching.

■ Build relationships with students. Interviews with African-American high school students who presented behavior challenges for staff revealed that they wanted their teachers to discover what their lives were like outside of school and that they wanted an opportunity to partake in the school's reward systems. Developing an understanding of students' lives also enables the teacher to increase the relevance of lessons and make examples more meaningful.

■ De Anne Wellman-Owre, an SLP practicing in Rhode Island, encouraged SLPs to "attempt to communicate with and get to know family members in order to gain insight into cultural barriers that might impact the child's learning. Help the family to adjust their expectations of school and their child's learning experiences and performance" (D. Wellman-Owre, personal communication, August 1, 2005).

■ Focus on the ways students learn and observe students to identify their task orientations. Once students' orientations are known, the teacher can structure tasks to take them into account. For example, some students may need time to prepare or attend to details before they can begin a task, they. For these students, the teacher can allow time for students to prepare, provide them with advance organizers, and announce how much time will be given for preparation and when the task will begin. This is a positive way to honor their need for preparation, rituals, or customs. Payne (1998a, 1988b) offered some good resources to use in implementing this approach. SLPs practicing in Wisconsin public schools have used Payne's information to learn how to effectively use clinical strategies such as visuals,

concrete organizers, and timelines (M. Jagodzinski, personal communication, August 20, 2005).

■ Teach students to match their behaviors to the setting. People behave differently in different settings. For example, more formal behavior is the norm at official ceremonies. Teaching students the differences among their home, school, and community settings can help them switch to appropriate behavior for each context. For example, the SLP may describe the differences between conversations with friends in the community and conversations with adults at school and confirm that each behavior is valued and useful in that setting. Although some students adjust their behavior automatically, others must be taught and provided ample opportunities to practice. Involving families and the community can help students learn to adjust their behavior in each of the settings in which they interact.

Burnette (1999) also offered some *instructional strategies* for improving the teaching-learning relationship with culturally diverse students:

■ Use a variety of instructional strategies and learning activities. Offering variety provides students with opportunities to learn in ways that are responsive to their own communication styles, cognitive styles, and aptitudes. In addition, the variety helps them develop and strengthen other approaches to learning.

■ Consider students' cultures and language skills when developing learning objectives and instructional activities. Facilitate comparable learning opportunities for students with differing characteristics. It is important to consider that students may differ in appearance, race, sex, disability, ethnicity, religion, socioeconomic status, or ability.

■ Incorporate objectives for affective and personal development. Provide increased opportunities for high and low achievers to boost their self-esteem, develop positive self-attributes, and enhance their strengths and talents. Such opportunities can enhance students' motivation to learn and achieve. For example, a low-achieving high school student can be recruited to serve as a tutor for younger students.

- Communicate expectations. Let the students know the "classroom rules" about talking, verbal participation in lessons, and moving about the room. Tell them how long a task will take to complete or how long it will take to learn a skill or strategy, and when appropriate, give them information on their ability to master a certain skill or complete a task. For example, it may be necessary to encourage students who expect to achieve mastery but are struggling to do so. They may need to know that they have the ability to achieve mastery, but must work through the difficulty.

- Provide rationales. Explain the benefits of learning a concept, skill, or task. Ask students to identify the rationale for learning, and explain how the concept or skill applies to their lives at school, home, and work.

- Use advance and "post" organizers. At the beginning of lessons, give the students an overview and tell them the purpose or goal of the activity. If applicable, tell them the order that the lesson will follow and relate it to previous lessons. At the end of the lesson, summarize its main points.

- Provide frequent reviews of the content learned. For example, check with the student to see if they remember the difference between simple and compound sentences. Provide a brief review of the previous lesson before continuing on to a new and related lesson.

- Facilitate independence in thinking and action. Teachers can use many different ways to facilitate students' independence. For example, when students ask questions, the teacher can encourage independence by responding in a way that lets students know how to find the answer for themselves. When teachers ask students to evaluate their own work or progress, they are facilitating independence, and asking students to perform for the class (e.g., by reciting or role playing) also promotes independence.

- Promote student on-task behavior. Keeping students on-task maintains a high level of intensity of instruction. By starting lessons promptly and minimizing transition time between lessons, teachers can help students stay on-task. Shifting smoothly (no halts) and efficiently (no wasted effort) from one lesson to another and being efficient about housekeeping tasks such as handing out papers and setting up audiovisual equipment will help to maintain their attention. Keeping students actively involved in the lessons—for example, by asking questions that require students to recall information—also helps them to stay focused and increases the intensity of instruction.

- Monitor students' academic progress during lessons and independent work. Check with students during seatwork to see if they need assistance before they have to ask for help. Ask if they have any questions about what they are doing and if they understand what they are doing. Also make the students aware of the various situations in which a skill or strategy can be used as well as adaptations that will broaden its applicability to additional situations.

- Provide frequent feedback. Feedback at multiple levels is preferred. For example, acknowledging a correct response is a form of brief feedback, while prompting a student who has given an incorrect answer by providing clues or repeating or rephrasing the question constitutes feedback at another level. The teacher also may give positive feedback by stating the appropriate aspects of the student's performance. Finally, the teacher may give positive corrective feedback by making students aware of specific aspects of their performance that need work, reviewing concepts and asking questions, making suggestions for improvement, and having the students correct their work.

■ Require mastery. Ensure that students master one task before going on to the next. When tasks are assigned, tell the students the criteria that define mastery and the different ways in which mastery can be attained. When mastery is achieved on one aspect or portion of the task, give students corrective feedback to let them know what aspects they have mastered and what aspects still need more work. When the task is complete, let the students know that mastery was reached.

Many of the foregoing strategies may be applicable to all students, regardless of their culture. They are really just good teaching strategies.

Cultural Competence Related to Curriculum Content and Intervention

SLPs must write IEP goals that are curriculum based. Therefore, SLPs need to know the curriculum standards and how to incorporate general education materials into the intervention process. State curriculum standards typically include information related to the history and culture of various ethnic groups. Leary (1998, 2004) provided examples The SLP must become culturally competent and also must help students become culturally competent. Four approaches toward that end were defined by Banks (1993) and described by Vaughn, Boss, and Schumm (1997). These approaches are summarized next:

■ *Contributions approach.* Ethnic heroes and cultural artifacts are added to the curriculum content.
■ *Additive approach.* The basic content of the curriculum remains the same and added content, concepts, themes, and perspectives that focus on diversity are introduced.
■ *Transformation approach.* The basic curriculum is changed, and all events, concepts, and themes are considered from multiple perspectives based on diversity.
■ *Social action approach.* The transformation approach is taken one step further, and a problem-solving process is used to help students make decisions and take actions related to the concept, issue, or problem being studied. The problem- solving activities involve three steps: (1) identify the problem or questions; (2) collect data related to the problem or question; and (3) conduct a value inquiry and analysis.

For example, the students may identify discrimination in school as the problem. They identify concrete examples of discrimination and discuss the causes. Finally, they examine and reflect on their own values, attitudes, and beliefs related to discrimination.

Summary

The school-based SLP must consider cultural competency as related to all aspects of the professional scope of practice including prevention, assessment/evaluation, intervention, managerial style, interpersonal skills, advocacy, and supervision. Developing cultural competence is an ethical responsibility, as well as a legal mandate. IDEA '04 set forth the mandate that each child is entitled to a complete assessment and evaluation process that is nondiscriminatory. New assessment tools and procedures that address cultural differences must be explored. The SLP needs to collaborate with other educators when developing curriculum-based IEPs. The SLP must be aware of unique mandates related to cultural issues in the state where he or she practices. The SLP must collaborate with others to create a school climate where every individual is valued.

Questions for Application and Review

1. What are some typical reactions to unfamiliar cultures?
2. Paraphrase the seven strategies that Battle describes as helpful in learning to become culturally competent.
3. What are some ways in which African-American cultures differ from other cultures?
4. What are some attitudes held by persons of Asian-American cultures that differ from the typical classroom expectations?
5. What is meant by *basic interactive competency skill*?
6. What is meant by *cognitive academic language proficiency*?
7. Why do school-based SLPs need to take into consideration the difference between BICS and CALP when conducting classroom observations?
8. What are some pitfalls of using standardized tests with students from diverse cultures?
9. Describe three alternative assessment approaches that may be used in place of standardized tests for assessing the communication skills of students from diverse cultures?
10. Why is it important for SLPs to know the history, culture, and heritage of the people of their state?

References

Adler, S. (1993). *Multicultural communication skills in the classroom*. Needham Heights, MA: Allyn & Bacon.

American Speech-Language-Hearing Association. (2003). *Code of ethics*. Available at http://www.asha.org/policy

American Speech-Language-Hearing Association. (2004). Definition of communication disorders and variations. *The ASHA Leader, 35*(Suppl. 10), 40–41.

American Speech-Language Hearing Association. (2007). *Directory of speech-language pathology assessment instruments: VI. Evaluation tool for culturally and linguistically diverse populations*. Available at http://www.asha.org/policy

Banks, J. A. (1993). Approaches to multicultural curriculum reform. In J. A. Banks (Ed.), *Multicultural education: Issues and perspectives* (2nd ed., pp. 208–209). Boston: Allyn & Bacon.

Battle, D. (1998). *Communication disorders in multicultural populations* (2nd ed.). Newton, MA: Butterworth-Heinemann.

Bishop, S. (1988). *Identification of language disorders in Vietnamese children*. Unpublished master's thesis, San Diego State University, San Diego, CA.

Bloom, B. S. (1956). *Taxonomy of educational objectives: The classification of educational goals*. New York: David McKay.

Burnette, J. (1999). Critical behaviors and strategies for teaching culturally diverse students. *ERIC Digest*, EDO-99-12.

Cheng, L. (1991). *Assessing Asian language performance: Guidelines for evaluating limited-English proficient students*. Oceanside, CA: Academic Communication Associates.

Cheng, L. (1999a). Many voices, many tongues: Accents, dialects, and variations: forward. *Topics in Language Disorders, 19*(4), vi.

Cheng, L. (1999b). Moving beyond accent: Social and cultural realities of living with many tongues. *Topics in Language Disorders, 19*, 4–7.

Crago, M. B. (1992). Ethnography and language socialization: A cross-cultural perspective. *Topics in Language Disorders, 12*, 28–39.

Crais, E. (1994, April). Birth to three: Current assessment tools and techniques. Short course presented at the annual conference of the Tennessee Association of Audiologists and Speech-Language Pathologists, Gatlinburg, TN.

Crais, E. (1995). Expanding the repertoire of tools and techniques for assessing communication skills of infants and toddlers. *American Journal of Speech-Language Pathology, 4*(3), 47–59.

Crowley, C. (2003). *Diagnosing communication disorders in culturally and linguistically diverse students*. (ERIC Document Reproduction Service No. E 650)

Crowley, C., & Valenti, D. (2004). Diagnosing communication disorders in children who are culturally and linguistically diverse. *Communication Connection, 18*(3), 1-3.

Cummins, J. (1984). *Bilingualism and special education: Issues in assessment and pedagogy*. San Diego, CA: College-Hill Press.

Dollaghan, C. (1985). Child meets word: "Fast mapping" in preschool children. *Journal of Speech and Hearing Research, 28*, 449-454.

Freiberg, C. (1997). *Linguistically culturally diverse populations: African American & Hmong*. Madison, WI: Wisconsin Department of Public Instruction.

Hall, E. (1976). *Beyond culture*. Garden City, NY: Doubleday/Anchor Press.

Harris, G. (1993). American Indian cultures: A lesson in diversity. In D. E. Battle (Ed.), *Communication disorders in multicultural populations*. Boston: Butterworth-Heinemann.

Heath, S. B. (1982). What no bedtime story means: Narrative skills at home and school. In *Language in Society, 2*, 49-76.

Hegde, M. N., & Davis, D. (1995). *Clinical methods and practicum in speech-language pathology* (2nd ed.). San Diego, CA: Singular.

Hofstede, G. T. (1991). *Cultures and organizations: Software of the mind*. London: McGraw Hill.

Hwa-Froelich, D. (2000). Play assessment for children from culturally and linguistically diverse backgrounds). *Language Learning and Education, 11*(2), 6-9.

Hwa-Froelich, D., Westby, C., & Schommer-Aikins, M. (December, 2000). Assessing language learnability. *Language Learning and Education, 7*(3), 3.

Leary, J. P. (1998). *American Indian studies program information packet*. Department of Public Instruction. Madison, Wisconsin.

Leary, J. P. (2004, December). *Act 31: Educational needs and provisions requiring the study of the history, culture, and tribal sovereignty of the federally-recognized tribes and bands in Wisconsin*. Presentation given at the University of Wisconsin, Madison, Wisconsin.

McCauley, R. J., & Swisher, L. (1984). Psychometric review of language and articulation tests for preschool children. *Journal of Speech and Hearing Disorders, 49*, 338-348.

McFadden, T. U. (1996). Creating language impairments in typically achieving children: The pitfalls of normal normative sampling. *Language, Speech, and Hearing Services in Schools, 27*, 3-9.

Oetting, J. B., Rice, M., & Swank, L. K. (1995). Quick incidental language learning (QUILL) of words by school-age children with and without SLI. *Journal of Speech and Hearing Research, 38*, 434-445.

Payne, R., K. (1998a). *A framework for understanding poverty modules 1-9 workbook*. Highlands, TX: Process.

Payne, R. K. (1998b). *Learning structures modules 10-16*. Highlands, TX: Process.

Pena, E., & Quinn, R. (1997). Task familiarity: Effects on the test performance of Puerto Rican and African-American children. *Language, Speech, and Hearing Services in School, 28*(4), 323-332.

Rice, M. L., Buhr, J. C., & Nemeth, M. (1990). Fast mapping word learning abilities of language delayed preschoolers. *Journal of Speech and Hearing Disorders, 55*, 33-42.

Rosin, R., & Gill, G. (1997, February). *Changing perspectives: Assessing your preadolescent children's communication skills: Implications for practicing clinicians*. Workshop presented at the University of Wisconsin, Madison, Wisconsin.

Schieffelin, B. B. (1994). Code-switching and language socialization. In J. F. Duchan, L. E. Hewitt, L. E. Sonnenmeier, & R. M. Sonnenmeier (Eds.), *Pragmatics: From theory to practice*. Englewood Cliffs, NJ: Prentice-Hall.

Schraeder, T., Quinn, M., Stockman, I., & Miller, J. (1999). Authentic assessment as an approach to preschool speech-language screening. *American Journal of Speech-Language Pathology, 8*(3), 195-200.

Taylor, O. (Ed). (1986). *Nature of communication disorders in culturally and linguistically diverse populations*. San Diego, CA: College-Hill Press.

Terrell, S. L., & Terrell, F. (1996). The importance of psychological and sociocultural factors for providing clinical services to African American children. In A. G. Kamhi, K. E. Pollock, & J. L. Harris (Eds.), *Communication development and disorders in African American children* (p. 55). Baltimore: Brookes.

Udvari, A., & Thousand, J. (1995). Promising practices that foster inclusive education. In R. Villa & J. Thousand (Eds.), *Creating an inclusive school* (p. 95). Alexandria, VA: Association for Supervision and Curriculum Development.

U.S. Census Bureau. (2000). *American community survey*. Data generated by Andrea Mosley using American Fact Finder. Retrieved May 21, 2004, from http://factfinder.census.gov/home/saff/main.html

Varner, I., & Beamer, L. (1995). *Intercultural communication in the global workplace*. Chicago: Irwin.

Vaughn, S., Boss, C., & Schumm, J. (1997). *Teaching mainstreamed diverse, and at-risk students in the general education classroom*. Needham Heights, MA: Allyn & Bacon.

Westby, C. E. (2000). A scale for assessing development of children's play. In C. Schaefer, K. Gilpin, & A. Sandrine (Eds.), *Play diagnosis and assessment* (2nd ed., pp. 15–57). New York: Wiley.

Wetherby, A., & Prizant, B. (1992). Profiling your children's communicative competence. In S. Warren & J. Riechle (Eds.), *Causes and effects in communication and language intervention* (pp. 217–253). Baltimore: Brookes.

Wolfram, W. (1976). Sociolinguistic levels of test bias. In T. Trabasso & D. Harrison (Eds.), *Seminar in Black English* (pp. 265–267). Mahwah, NJ: Erlbaum.

Zentella, A. C. (1997). *Growing up bilingual: Puerto Rican children in New York*. Malden, MA: Blackwell.

Chapter 8

CONFERENCING, COUNSELING, AND CREATING A SENSE OF COMMUNITY

RELATED VOCABULARY

advice shopping   The process of seeking information from a variety of sources until one hears what is most pleasing or expected.

information-gathering conference   A type of conference in which the professional seeks out information that is only known to the parent or legal guardian.

introductory conference   A type of conference with the primary purpose of establishing a cooperative feeling, trust, and open communication.

listening post   The process of seeking out another person who will listen to whatever one wishes to discuss, whether or not it is relevant to the educational setting.

problem-solving conference   A type of conference in which the school representatives share what has been tried, what the outcomes have been, what has not been accomplished, and what needs to be accomplished and then engages the parents or legal guardian in a brainstorming activity to identify possible solutions.

reporting conference   A type of conference in which the school representative shares specific information about a student's program, progress, products, strengths, challenges, interests, learning style, behavioral needs, behavioral expectations, goals, or aspirations.

unscheduled drop-in   A visit from a parent or legal guardian who does not have an appointment, catches the educator at an inopportune time, and expects to have a conference immediately.

Introduction

The modern-day speech-language pathologist (SLP) must become a member of the collaborative educational team that creates the school culture. Gone are the days when the school-based SLP could slip in and out of several schools providing itinerant services in isolated settings. As stated by Judy Rudebusch, an SLP active in professional research and policy making, "The SLP of yesterday may have said, 'I work at a school and I have a caseload of 40 children,' but the modern-day SLP must say, 'I work at a school and I am a part of the school community that supports a positive learning atmosphere for all children, not just the children on my caseload'" (J. Rudebusch, statement during a discussion at an ASHA ad hoc committee meeting, July 2002).

The Child Development Project (CDP, 1994) advocated that schools must foster caring relationships, not only in the classroom but also on the playground and throughout the school building. Creating a *sense of community* is the first step toward positive relationships. The SLP who does not have time in his or her workload devoted to creating a sense of community might as well relinquish all other efforts related to conferencing and counseling. Without trust and caring relationships, effective counseling and conferencing will not happen. Trust must be established between the SLP and other educators; between the SLP and administrators; between the SLP and parents, legal guardians, or caregivers; and between the SLP and students.

The CDP (1994) documented that schoolwide activities may either reinforce or undermine initiatives to develop trust. The best way to facilitate trust is to create activities that are inclusive, support children's learning, foster an appreciation of differences, and provide children with the opportunity to help others. The five essential community-building ingredients identified by the CDP can be summarized as follows.

1. *Inclusion and participation.* All parents, students, and school staff members should be invited to participate freely in schoolwide activities, particularly those designed for families, whether traditional or nontraditional, to enjoy together. The invitations must be warm, welcoming, and nonthreatening. The activities must be designed with attention to special language, cultural, economic, and child care needs of the participating families.

2. *Cooperative environment.* Students and families should be able to enjoy cooperative, noncompetitive activities that promote the value of learning together and helping others. Everyone should feel good about succeeding. The activities should not create "losers."

3. *Emphasis on responsibility and helpfulness.* Students should be given opportunities to experience the value of helping others. Everyone should take responsibility within and outside of the school community.

4. *Appreciation of differences.* Parents, students, and school staff members should be made to feel that their social and cultural backgrounds are valued and respected within the school community. Everyone should share his or her cultural heritage and learn from others.

5. *Reflection.* Everyone should be encouraged to reflect on what has been learned from the group experience and from working together.

When a family identifies with the school, feels included, feels appreciated, and has participated in a cooperative environment that has fostered a sense of responsibility and helpfulness, the doors of communication will be open when the need for conferencing or counseling arises. When a family does not identify with the school, has not felt included, has felt cultural alienation, and has been made to feel incompetent in some way, the doors of communication may quickly slam shut.

Creating a Positive First Contact

It is essential that the first contact between the SLP and parent, legal guardian, or caregiver be a positive one. In the past, many schools held open house nights as a way for professionals and parents to come together in a nonthreatening, positive first encounter. Some schools have transformed the traditional open house night from the "show and tell–walk through–eat cookies" scenario into a more interactive, "fun" activity. When children can see that their parents are interested in what they are learning and how they are learning it, they become more eager students and more willing to participate (CDP, 1994). Some innovative, collaborative community-building activities include holding a family film night, family read-aloud fest, science night, math night, family sing-out, or dance night; creating a schoolwide mural, community garden, or family heritage museum; and conducting a fundraiser for a worthy cause. All of these alternatives are not competitive. An illuminating example is the contrast between a traditional science fair and a noncompetitive family fun night that focuses on science learning. The noncompetitive family fun night provides all participants with a collaborative experience that creates a sense of belonging and caring. The differences between a traditional science fair and a science family fun night are shown in Table 8–1.

School-based SLPs should know about these different approaches to collaborative team build-

ing. They are among the professionals who most frequently engage in conferencing and counseling with a student or family. Thus, SLPs have a stake in building a trust relationship through schoolwide activities that develop a community of caring.

Tips and Techniques for Parent-Teacher Conferences and Individual Education Program Meetings

IDEA '04 mandated that progress related to a student's individualized education program (IEP) must be reported at least as often as general education progress reports are given. For example, if report cards are given on a quarterly basis, then IEP progress must be reported on a quarterly basis. If report cards are given on a trimester schedule, then IEP progress must be reported each trimester. IDEA '04 also placed more emphasis on providing services in a least restrictive environment. As a result, SLPs are finding a greater need to collaborate with other educators during parent-teacher conferences.

Although IDEA '04 required that IEP progress be reported as frequently as general education reports progress, each local school district determines

Table 8–1. Comparison of Traditional Science Fair and Noncompetitive Family Science Night

Characteristic	Traditional Science Fair	Science Family Fun Night
Purposes	Individual student projects are displayed; students and families view the projects; awards or ribbons are given to the outstanding projects	Learning stations are created; students and families visit each station and complete an activity together; everyone celebrates one another's successes
Goals	Competitive; goal is to win; some people win, others lose	Collaborative; goal is to participate; everyone wins, no one loses
Student participation	Students work individually	Students work with families and other students
Parent and educator participation	Parents observe; educators judge	Parents participate; educators participate
Inclusion/exclusion factor	Excludes students and families who are unwilling to compete	Includes everyone

Source: Child Development Project, (1994).

how parents are kept informed of their student's progress. Many different formats are used:

- Some school districts keep the IEP reporting process separate from the classroom report card process even though they both follow the same schedule of frequency.
- Some school districts send home written IEP progress notes and report cards twice a year and hold face-to-face parent-teacher conferences and separate face-to-face IEP progress conferences twice a year.
- Some school districts use a portfolio system. Individualized conferences are held with each student's parents three or four times per year. Progress reports related to the IEP may or may not be included in the portfolio reporting system.
- Some school districts combine the report card and IEP progress report into one collaborative system. The general educator and a member of the child's IEP team meet with the parents and discuss progress related to all of the student's educational services.
- Some school districts hold teleconferences or videoconferences with parents.

These are just a few of the ways in which school districts maintain control over their local school system. The mandates may be met in many different ways. The mandated annual IEP meeting also is different from the IEP progress report system.

Some general guidelines relevant to parent-teacher conferences are relevant for all educators. Before parent conferencing is undertaken, it is important to remember the "four Ps": *prior, proper planning is paramount!* At least six other Ps are recognized as necessary for effective conferencing:

- *Prepared.* Have a vision. What is the expected outcome of the parent conference? Is the conference expected to achieve a directive, a recommendation, a compromise, a majority vote, or a consensus? Visualizing the outcome of

the conference and preparing accordingly are important. All materials (whether test scores, informal classroom observation checklists, written testimonials, samples of the student's work, audiotape, videotape, or computer software) should be well organized and easily accessible. The SLP should know what key bits of information must be conveyed and how to make them understood. The support of other professionals, when appropriate, can be enlisted.

- *Punctual.* The SLP should arrive a few minutes early so that he or she does not feel rushed, nervous, or harried. The SLP should be able to offer a warm, welcoming, relaxed greeting.
- *Polite.* It is best to err on the side of conservatism. First names should not be used unless the person has given permission to do so. The SLP should know the correct last names of each person involved. In today's blended family structures, it is not unusual for a mother, father, student, and sibling to have different last names. Another important consideration is the cultural customs related to the use of the family name.
- *Professional.* Wearing casual-business clothing, maintaining a respectful demeanor, and knowing the cultural customs related to pragmatics will help identify the SLP as a capable professional.
- *Positive.* The SLP should always begin the conference on a positive note. In discussing the student's strengths, challenges, interests, and learning style, it is best to begin with the strengths.
- *Persistent.* If a parent, legal guardian, or caregiver does not show up for an appointment or a scheduled conference, it should be rescheduled. The school should make at least three good-faith efforts. IDEA '04 allows parents, legal guardians, or caregivers to participate in IEP conferences via several options, including videoconferencing and teleconferencing modes. Conducting a

home visit is another option. Be sure to offer these, if needed.

At the start of any conference, a mutually agreeable objective should be clearly stated. Otherwise, the conference may proceed as two parallel conversations in which neither party appears to be listening to the other. A clearly stated conference goal could be framed as follows: "I'm delighted that you were able to meet with me today so that we may discuss Janet's home carryover program for her articulation goals." When differing objectives are evident, Hunter (1978) documented that the SLP has three choices: (1) focus on the original objective and make another appointment to address the other concern; (2) identify the two different objectives and allow the parent, legal guardian, or caregiver to choose which one to address; or (3) accept the alternative objective. Every conference should have an agreed-on objective that is clear to all parties involved.

Hunter (1978) identified four different types of parent-teacher conferences that may be held: the introductory conference, the reporting conference, the information-gathering conference, and the problem-solving conference. Tips for maximizing the benefit from each type of conference offered by Hunter are summarized next.

Introductory Conference

When conducting an **introductory conference**, it is important to allow sufficient notification time. At least 2 weeks' notice should be provided. Parents, legal guardians, or caregivers may need to make child care arrangements for siblings, transportation arrangements, or work schedule arrangements. It is not realistic to schedule a conference within a few days of notification. The SLP may be wise to enlist the services of a high school student or other volunteer who is ready to provide child care for siblings who unexpectedly accompany the parent, legal guardian, or caregiver to the conference. During an introductory conference, the SLP must consider what information to include or exclude. The purpose of an introductory conference is to have a positive first contact and establish rapport. Thus, more "difficult" information may best be given at a future conference, while this conference focuses on the student's strengths, interests, and learning style. The introductory conference should last no more than 30 minutes. The SLP should offer concrete examples and descriptions of the student's work and know how to graciously end on time.

Reporting Conference

The **reporting conference** is the occasion for more in-depth discussion of a student's previously identified challenges or behavioral issues. When preparing for a reporting conference, the SLP should consult with other educators and find out if anyone else is facing similar issues. A collaborative team conference may be most appropriate. The SLP must determine what information should be given and have that information carefully organized and readily available. The SLP also should determine how or if the student will participate. The student may not be physically present at the conference but instead write a letter to his or her parents, guardians, or caregivers that will be read at the conference. The student may be physically present only during the first or last half of the conference. Under these conditions, the SLP has time to involve the student in the discussion and also time to interact without the student present. Another alternative is to have the student present but, as agreed beforehand, only as a listener or only to talk about the issues of concern. The SLP is wise to do prior, proper planning when determining the optimal interaction scenario for the benefit of the student.

Information-Gathering Conference

The **information-gathering conference** is one in which parents, legal guardians, or caregivers provide the information. For example, the purpose of this type of conference may be to collect health and developmental history information. The SLP should prepare by gathering descriptive data and formulating relevant questions. The SLP should begin by stating the problem with concern and tact. Appropriate measures to ensure confidentiality are identified. The SLP ends the conference by thanking the parents, legal guardians, or caregivers, letting them know how useful the information has been, and assuring them that the information will be held confidential and used in the best interest of the student.

Problem-Solving Conference

For a **problem-solving conference**, the SLP must provide concrete examples of what the school has done, what the results have been, what the school cannot do, and what the parents can do to help. Using the phrase "I need your help" is a door opener during a problem-solving conference. The SLP also needs to find out how well equipped a parent, legal guardian, or caregiver is to help. For example, the single mother who is working two jobs may not realistically be able to conduct a home carryover program. Thus, the SLP also must determine ways to support the student's communication program at home. For example, perhaps the help of a college student or senior citizen currently volunteering with the after-school program would be a workable option for conducting the carryover program.

During the problem-solving conference, a definition of success related to the specific outcome must be clearly understood by all parties. For example, at a particular point in the student's program, if the SLP considers production of /s/ clusters at the sentence level as a successful target behavior, rather than production of /s/ in all positions at the conversation level, then that difference must be clearly communicated.

Canter and Canter (1985) described five different emotional patterns that may not be productive and may surface during a conference:

- **Advice shopping**
- Reluctance
- Seeking a **listening post**
- **Unscheduled drop-in**
- Anger

To a certain extent, these five scenarios represent the five characteristics of grieving identified by

Gough (2004): denial, depression, anger, guilt, and fear.

Parents Who May Be "Advice Shopping"

A parent who is "advice shopping" may exemplify a person who is in denial that a disability actually exists. Gough (2004) provided a poignant rationale for denial as a function of buying time until the person is able to identify external and internal supports so that he or she may begin to face the reality. As described by Gough, denial may serve as a series of "floodgates" to prevent the affected person from "drowning in sorrow." At a certain point, the first and highest set of floodgates opens, and the water rushes to come to the top of the next set of gates. Some water splashes over and is absorbed into the ground, but a major flood is prevented at that time. Bit by bit, each set of floodgates opens until the person is able to cope with the flood waters. Denial allows the person to continue to function and deal with what needs to be done (e.g., paying the mortgage, feeding the children) and serves as the first step in the process of grieving.

"Advice shoppers" go from professional to professional in hopes of finding the one who will tell them what they want to hear. These parents have had their child or adolescent evaluated by every possible clinic and private practitioner but are still not ready to accept the diagnosis ascribed. When dealing with the advice shopper, it is important to find out what the parents have already tried. The SLP should have the parent sign a release of information form and ask that all relevant reports be sent before the face-to-face conference; any questions will need to be clarified. The SLP should not conduct the conference alone; another educator, the local education agency (LEA) representative, or an administrator should be present. It is appropriate to give some degree of emotional support (e.g., "I know how difficult this is for you; I know how hard you've tried"). The needs of the parent should be assessed, but it is important to stay within the SLP's scope of practice set forth by ASHA (2001). The SLP should not serve as the primary counselor who assists the parent through the grieving process. During a conference with a parent who is advice shopping, plenty of tissues should be within reach for the parent's use. Emotions often run high, even when the session is positive.

Parents Who May Be Reluctant

A reluctant parent may exemplify a person who is experiencing depression or fear. Gough (2004) reported that a person's sense of self-worth that was developed within the context of family, culture, and an era often is challenged severely by issues of loss, particularly disability. Facing a disability shakes a person's sense of feeling competent, strong, and valuable. Most parents would rather experience an illness, pain, or disability themselves before wishing it on their children, so the degree of depression and fear faced by a parent of a child with a disability can be overwhelming.

The reluctant parent often has not had a positive school experience when he or she was younger. Accordingly, such parents rarely attend schoolwide functions, often cancel meetings, and sometimes fail to show up for conferences and meetings. In dealing with a reluctant parent, it is essential that the first contact be a positive one. The SLP may consider offering a videoconference, teleconference, or home visit as an alternative to a school meeting. In making a home visit, it is recommended that at least one other educator or professional accompany the SLP. If the parent does actually come into the school for the conference, the SLP should make every effort to help the parent feel comfortable. Helpful measures may include having an interpreter present, honoring social rituals from the family's culture, bringing in adult-size chairs and an adult-size table for the purpose of the conference, and moving to a room that has such accommodations. Such measures may make a significant difference to the reluctant parent.

Parents Who May Be Seeking a Listening Post

A parent or other caregiver who wants to use the SLP as a listening post may exemplify someone who is experiencing guilt. The person seems to want to talk and talk, as though on a daunting quest to answer the question *why?* Gough (2004) explained that guilt drives this exploration of responsibility for the loss. Guilt is related to one's personal belief system about power and causality in the universe. Gough ascertained that a person cannot be talked out of guilt. It takes an intensive process of dialogue with a trusted person to overcome guilt.

The parent seeking a listening post talks continuously and never seems to need to take a breath. The person may go off on tangents and introduce topics completely unrelated to the objective of the conference. Such parents, if given the SLP's home phone number, may call every night, to talk and talk. When dealing with such a parent, each professional must set his or her own boundaries. Is the SLP comfortable giving out a home phone number? Is the SLP willing to spend additional hours during the evening and weekends listening to a parent? This is a policy that all such professionals must prepare for in advance. It is essential that the SLP stay within the scope of practice (i.e., recognize the limits of his or her expertise). It may be necessary to cut the "listening post" parent short before he or she reveals confidential information that may not be appropriate (such as marital problems) and to provide a gentle reminder about focusing on the conference objective. A possible response in such cases might be: "I hear that you are troubled, but I am not the best person to help you. I have too much respect for the complexities of your issues to try to help you by myself." The SLP should keep a directory of relevant, qualified professionals so that the parent may be referred to a licensed social worker, counselor, psychologist, or psychiatrist.

Parents Who Appear to Be Angry

The anger that a person feels internally may be projected onto the professional who is the bearer of bad news. Gough (2004) recommended exploring the anger, rather than trying to calm, avoid, distract, or redirect it. Smart (2001) explained that sometimes the anger springs from deep-rooted prejudices and discrimination related to disabilities. In the English language the prefixes *dis* and *dys* mean difficult, impaired, or absent. Words such as *disorders, disability, disease, dyslexia, dystrophy,* and *dysfunction* reflect these meanings. The prefixes *im-* and *in-* mean absence or lack of; therefore, the word *invalid* means without value or validity; *impairment* means without strength or quality (i.e., spoiled); and *infirm* means without strength. Thus, most people without disabilities think of a disability as a deficit or sign of inferiority. A person whose child is diagnosed with a disability may have deep-rooted stereotypes or prejudices. When the person learns that the child has been diagnosed with a disability, those deeply rooted feelings of prejudices and discrimination may evolve into feelings of anger. The person may be feeling, "Not my child!"

The SLP should not meet with an angry parent alone. Other educators or professionals, the LEA representative, or an administrator should be present. In dealing with the angry parent, one strategy is to listen without saying anything. When the parent has finished, the SLP should allow a 10- to 15- second pause time of complete silence. In that time, the parent may pull himself or herself together and actually apologize for the anger. On the other hand, the person's anger may escalate because he or she is frustrated by the lack of response. Another strategy is to verbally acknowledge the parent's anger. This verbal validation sometimes diffuses the emotion. Sharing the SLP's own feelings with the parent, without becoming overtly emotional, sometimes helps (e.g., "I feel uncomfortable when you raise your voice and use profanity"). Sometimes it is necessary to stop the conference and reschedule it for another time.

Parents Who Make an Unscheduled Drop-in Visit

The SLP must be wary of the "unscheduled drop-in." A concerned parent may stop the SLP at the entrance of the school, in the aisle of the grocery store or the line at the post office, or at an evening schoolwide function with the intent of holding a conference right there on the spot. The SLP should not hold parent conferences without prior, proper planning or in a location that does not ensure privacy and confidentiality. The only exception may be in the case of an emergency or perhaps the first overture of a reluctant parent.

Other Considerations in Parent-Teacher Conferences

Learning about a disorder may be accompanied by shock even if the diagnosis is anticipated. Thus, in parent-teacher conferences, kindness, sensitivity, and common sense take precedence over technical information. The professional must be considerate of the myriad emotions that a parent, legal guardian, or caregiver may experience during a conference when an initial diagnosis is made. Schum (1986) identified confusion, anxiety, frustration, hostility, loss, depression, anger, fear, denial, displacement, reaction formation, projection, avoidance, rationalization, and intellectualization as possible reactions. Margolis (2004) documented that people typically remember approximately 25% of what they have been told in a conference. This may be due in part to the internal highly emotional state of the person, even if he or she appears calm externally. Professionals may become desensitized over time because they have dealt with so many conferences throughout their careers. For the parent, legal guardian, or caregiver, however, the conference is a new experience. Thus, parents, legal guardians, or caregivers attending the conference may be operating on an entirely different plane of emotions from that for the professionals involved. Writing a follow-up letter after the conference, maintaining a copy of the letter, and sending the original to the parent, legal guardian, or caregiver by mail is an important strategy. It will help clarify the information that may have been lost in a sea of hidden emotions experienced during the conference.

Student Records and Confidentiality

The SLP should know the legal aspects of accessing, creating, and using student records. State and federal statutes related to student records and confidentiality must be honored by all school districts and must be part of the knowledge base of all professionals in the school setting. School districts that use electronic billing for Medicaid reimbursement must comply with the Health Insurance Portability and Accountability Act of 1996. "A major goal of the Privacy Rule is to assure [sic] that individuals' health information is properly protected while allowing the flow of health information needed to provide and promote high quality health care and to protect the public's health and well being" (U.S. Department of Health and Human Services, 2003). The Family Educational Rights and Privacy Act (FERPA, 1974) is the federal law that applies to school records and outlines the requirements of educational recordkeeping. FERPA mandated that every school district must have written educational records and that personally identifiable information about students must be kept confidential. Parents have the right to inspect and review such records and also have the right to request copies. When a school staff member views confidential records, an access log must be kept. The access record must identify the staff member by name and title. Parents must consent before information from confidential records is shared with outside agencies or other professionals. Parents may request an amendment of records if they consider the information to be inaccurate or misleading. Notes retained by a staff member that are not shared with anyone else are not considered part of the confidential record.

When a student turns 18 years old, parents may no longer access a student's records unless that student provides permission. Educational records do not include treatment records of students 18 years or older that are maintained by health care professionals. Every public school district is required to adopt an educational records policy and to implement procedures that meet the standards of the FERPA. The school district must notify parents and students of their rights pertaining to student records, maintain a permanent file on each student, and maintain separate special education records. Parents have the right to refuse disclosure of directory information to the public. Each state may enact its own local law.

When a discrepancy exists between federal and state mandates, the more restrictive statute must be followed (Wisconsin Department of Public Instruction, 2004).

The types of records kept by a school district may include directory data, progress records, behavioral records, pupil physical health records, and patient health care records. School districts must have written policies about where each type of record is housed, who may access the information, and how the information is used. Descriptions of these types of record are provided next.

- *Directory data*—Records that include the student's name, address, telephone number, email address, date of birth, place of birth, weight, height, dates of attendance, photographs, name of the school most recently previously attended, and participation in extracurricular activities are all types of directory data. Directory data usually are more accessible to a wider audience within the school district.
- *Progress records*—Records that include the pupil's grades, attendance, immunization, screening results, and possibly extracurricular activities are types of progress records.
- *Behavioral records*—Records that include psychological test results, personality evaluations, documentation or summaries of conversations, written statements relating to the student's behavior, achievement test results, and physical health records are types of behavioral records. Such records often are kept in a separate file, in a separate file cabinet, and in a different location from that for directory data. Many school districts have policies that limit the personnel who have access to behavioral records.
- *Pupil physical health records*—Records that include basic health information about a student, including immunization records, an emergency medical card, a

log of first aid and medicine administered to the student, an athletic permit card, logs related to attendance of services provided by a physical or an occupational therapist, and documentation related to hearing, vision, scoliosis, and lead poisoning screenings, are types of pupil physical health records. Information such as diagnoses, opinion, and judgments made by a health care provider is not included in a physical health care record. Only basic health information may appear in such a file.

■ *Patient health care records*—Records relating to diagnoses, opinions, and judgments about a student made by a health care provider are examples of patient health care records. Written, drawn, printed, spoken, visual, electromagnetic, or digital information that is recorded or preserved must be kept in this separate file. IEP team summaries of evaluation findings, IEP team reports, IEP documents, intervention plans, remediation notes, and any other information that exceeds the definition of basic health information must be treated as a patient health care record.

Tips and Techniques for Personal Adjustment Counseling

Barrier, Li, and Jensen (2003) and Burroughs (2004) documented that discussion of the emotional aspects of a student's disorder may result in greater compliance with the intervention plan, greater satisfaction with intervention, increased rapport with the SLP, and better remediation outcomes. School-based SLPs must be trained in both informational counseling and personal adjustment counseling (Andrews, 2004; ASHA, 1997, 2001, 2003; Bloom & Cooperman, 2003; Margolis, 2004).

Informational counseling provides the student and family with the relevant information needed to understand the nature of the disorder and the steps that are recommended to manage it. Tetnowski (2003) pointed out that it is neces-

sary to provide accurate and unbiased information. Informational counseling is at the heart of the IEP process.

Personal adjustment counseling focuses on the emotional impact of the information (Margolis, 2004). Bloom and Cooperman (2003) described three stages of personal adjustment counseling. In stage I, the client tells his or her story through the use of the clinician-counselor's listening skills. In stage II, the clinician-counselor and client engage in active problem solving to help formulate goals and make desired changes. In stage III, the client "re-stories." New actions are taken, the goals are achieved, and the desired changes are made. This may sound like an easy process; however, it is one that the SLP may find most challenging and least prepared to execute. This section describes each stage in more detail.

Stage I: Let the Student's Story Unfold

Schneider (2003) explained that thoughts and feelings predate and dictate the content and form of children's verbal output and offers some counseling tips for the SLP who works with school-aged children. He offers these counseling strategies.

■ Begin the relationship by focusing on things that the student enjoys, knows well, and feels good about. Comment on things that are appreciated, respected, and admired about the student. When the relationship focuses on strengths, it can bolster overall self-confidence.

■ Let the student know that a good reason exists for each of his or her thoughts, feelings, and behaviors and that he or she is doing the best that is possible at the moment.

■ Acknowledge and validate the student's feelings, including those that are negative. This helps the student realize that feelings have a right to exist without being right or wrong.

■ Introduce strategies as options that can be employed in the future instead of pressuring the student to make changes he or she may not be ready for now. This sets the stage for the future and defines the place that the student may return to when he or she is ready.

■ Accept the student as he or she is in the present while believing in his or her potential for future growth.

■ Honor and respect the student's resistance to change. It is the student's active choice or will power that dictates what he or she will and will not do. This same active choice or will power is what will provide the fuel for later changes in the student.

Andrews (2004) offered five basic counseling techniques that the SLP may employ when guiding the student through stage I of the counseling process:

■ attending
■ empathy
■ unconditional positive regard
■ silence
■ neutral questioning

When the SLP is engaged in respectful *attending*, he or she is able to abandon his or her personal issues in order to understand the student's frame of reference. Respectful attending leads to empathy. When the SLP has achieved *empathy*, he or she is in tune with the student's needs. Some students are easy to work with and sessions are pleasant. Other students harbor more negative behaviors and are more difficult to deal with, so *unconditional positive regard* is harder to maintain. The SLP must learn to approach each session with curiosity and the desire to learn more about why the student feels the need to act out. *Silence* can be very powerful. Silence gives the student time to process and reflect on new information. Silence often gives the student a chance to express his or her own true feelings. SLPs are encouraged to audio- or videotape a session and analyze it based on the amount of student talk versus SLP talk after a period of silence. The SLP may be surprised by how much actual student communication may be achieved simply by employing silence. *Neutral questioning* also is effective because it is nonjudgmental. Neutral questions tend to be more open, rather than closed. Closed questions generally yield a "yes" or "no" answer whereas open questions give the student an opportunity to share what he or she is actually thinking or feeling.

Stage II: Engage in Active Problem Solving

Ouellette (2004) described solution-focused concepts that help the SLP bring the student into the second stage of counseling, active problem solving. Solution-focused therapy began in the 1970s with the work of Steve deShazer and InSoo Kim Berg. The model gained immense popularity and acceptance in the United States, Europe, and Asia.

Walter and Peller (1992) provided a brief overview of how solution-focused therapy works. First the clinician and the client define the desired outcome. Then the clinician helps the client focus on what is working, rather than focusing on what is not working. Finally, if the clinician sees that the client is doing something that is not working, he or she assists the client to replace that behavior with something that works better. The seven basic tenets of solution-focused therapy are summarized next:

1. Use of solution-oriented talk, rather than problem-oriented talk, is more effective.
2. Few problems exist all of the time; a focus on times when the problem does not happen or is less severe may lead to future solutions.
3. Change is continuous and ever-present.
4. Taking a very small first step will lead to larger subsequent steps.
5. Knowledge of how the student is able to work best can be used as a basis for building cooperation.
6. The clinician's role shifts from that of an expert to that of a consultant. The clinician observes what works best for the client and then uses professional expertise to build that solution into an effective clinical intervention that leads the student closer to the desired goal.
7. The family and the client have the best insights into how they go about solving problems and coping with difficult situations.

The SLP should make an effort to help students frame problem-solving efforts with a positive feeling tone. Jones (2003) offered several useful concepts: First, information can empower. Students can learn that information gained has a direct impact on life experiences. This concept may be shaped with such comments as "You are so smart about what your body is doing and how to make it change. That's something I am learning too— like when I get all stressed out; I can choose to relax." Second, understanding one's own uniqueness may be exciting. Third, learning to be a self-advocate can yield positive rewards. Fourth, learning to talk openly about a disability may create more confidence, and the child also will learn the benefits of sharing ideas. Fifth, connecting to people is important. Development of a support system can show a child what it is like to have a mentor. Sixth, persistence and patience can pay off. Finally, imperfection is human. By teaching these seven dispositions, the SLP can help the child learn to value overall communication skills, not just those based on speech production.

Stage III: New Actions

Once the student has had an opportunity to explore, express, and understand his or her emotions related to the communication delay or disorder and has engaged in active problem solving that is solution focused, he or she may be ready to take new actions to achieve the established goals. Involving the family may be the key to success. Research (Affleck, McGrade, McQueeney, & Allen, 1982; Casto & Mastropieri, 1986; Dunst, Trivette, & Cross, 1986; Guralnick, 1989; Nelson, 2004) has shown that family involvement consistently results in greater therapeutic success.

Nelson (2004) encouraged the use of the Self-Anchored Rating Scales (SARS) when working with family members. At the start of the program, SARS is introduced to the family as a scale of 0 to 10. Using the family's own language, a definition of the student's behavior at the start of the intervention program is used to anchor the scale. That description anchors the scale at point 0. At the opposite end is the family's description of the stu-

dent's behavior when intervention services are no longer needed. Then the family is asked to define changes that would move the student along the scale by one point or one-half point. Descriptors are created for each point on the scale. The construction of the scale helps define the program in objective, measurable terms. It also gives the parents, the student, and the SLP a common language so that they can communicate with each other more effectively. The family is asked to rate progress toward the goals. A solution-focused approach is used to find exceptions, discover effective strategies, evaluate efficacies, demonstrate competency, and provide encouragement. Hux (2003) offered some tips for working with families of persons with traumatic brain injury that may be applied to all families.

- Acknowledge that the family knows their loved one better than anyone else.
- Listen to their story.
- Have as a goal the following: "What can I learn from (not about) this family?"
- Understand how hope helps.
- Cry with the family; laugh with the family; show your human side.
- Talk to the family.
- Invite the family's involvement and know their concerns.
- Return phone calls promptly.
- Find out the family's best hope for the future.
- Recognize that the disability affects the family dynamics.
- Help the family find support groups of other families who are dealing with similar situations.

Summary

The SLP must become a part of the school culture and help create a caring community so that trust relationships with families may be nurtured. Positive first contacts lay the groundwork for later discussions that may be more difficult. When preparing for parent conferences and IEP meetings, the SLP needs to engage in prior, proper planning. The SLP should visualize the expected outcome; establish a positive, professional tone; and have relevant examples of the student's written work, verbal comments, and/or documented actions are readily available. The SLP needs to know how to use various conferencing formats and understand the difficult and varied emotions that may arise during a conference. The SLP should learn specific counseling strategies and know how to use them effectively. The SLP must learn how to work with families and how to maintain open communication.

Questions for Application and Review

1. Identify and describe five ingredients for creating a school climate that reflects a caring community.
2. Why is it important for the SLP to be an integral part of the school community?
3. What are the six Ps related to prior, proper planning for a parent conference or IEP meeting?
4. Describe an "advice-shopping" parent.
5. Describe a reluctant parent.
6. Describe a "listening post" parent.
7. Discuss the roots of anger that may surface when a parent learns that his or her child has been diagnosed with a disability.
8. Identify the three stages of counseling.
9. Discuss counseling strategies that are useful for the SLP.
10. Discuss important aspects of working with families.

References

Affleck, G., McGrade, B. J., McQueeney, M., & Allen, D. (1982). Promise of relationship-focused early intervention in developmental disabilities. *The Journal of Special Education, 16*(4), 413–430.

American Speech-Language-Hearing Association. (1997). *Preferred practice patterns for the profession of speech-language pathology.* Rockville, MD: Author.

American Speech-Language-Hearing Association. (2001). *Scope of practice, speech-language pathology.* Rockville, MD: Author.

American Speech-Language-Hearing Association. (2003). Code of ethics (revised). *ASHA, 23*(Suppl.), 13–15.

Andrews, M. (2004). Counseling techniques for speech-language pathologists. *Perspectives on Language and Education, 11*(1), 3–7.

Barrier, P., Li, J. T., & Jensen, N. M. (2003). Two words to improve physician-patient communication: What else? *Mayo Clinic Proceedings, 78,* 211–214.

Bloom, C., & Cooperman, D. (2003, December). Counseling and disorders of fluency: An overview. *Perspectives,* 207.

Burroughs, E. (2004). Encouraging the discussion of psychosocial issues. *Perspectives on Language Learning and Education, 11*(1), 25–26.

Canter, L., & Canter, M. (1985). *Assertive discipline.* Santa Monica, CA: Canter Associates.

Casto, G., & Mastropieri, M. A. (1986). The efficacy of early intervention programs: A meta-analysis. *Exceptional Children, 52*(5), 417–424.

Child Development Project. (1994). *At home in our schools.* Oakland, CA: Development Studies Center.

Dunst, C. J., Trivette, C. M., & Cross, A. H. (1986). Mediating influences of social support: Personal, family, and child outcomes. *American Journal of Mental Deficiency, 90,* 403–417.

Family Educational Rights and Privacy Act (FERPA). (1974). (20 U.S.C. § 1232g; 34 CFR Part 99).

Flahive, M. (2004, February). Counseling and the school-based speech-language pathologist. *ADVANCE for Speech-Language Pathologists & Audiologists,* 10–11.

Gough, D. (2004, March). Disability, loss, and grieving: Implications and suggestions for speech and language professionals. *Language Learning and Education, 11,* 18–25.

Guralnick, M. J. (1989). Recent developments in early intervention efficacy research: Implications for family involvement in P.L. 99-457. *Topics in Early Childhood Special Education, 9*(3), 1–17.

Hunter, M. (1978). *Effective parent conferences.* El Segundo, CA: TIP Publications.

Hux, K. (2003). *Assisting survivors of traumatic brain injury.* Austin, TX: Pro-Ed.

Jones, K. (2003, December). Counseling families: Life lessons. *Fluency and Fluency Disorders,* 17–20.

Margolis, R. (2004). What do your patients remember? *The Hearing Journal, 57*(6), 10–17.

Nelson, L. (2004). Using self-anchored rating scales in family-centered treatment. *Perspectives on Language Learning and Education, 11*(1), 14–17.

Ouellette, S. (2004). Applications of solution-focused concepts to the practice of speech-language pathology. *Perspectives on Language Learning and Education, 11*(1), 8–13.

Schneider, P. (2003, December). Counseling school-age children who stutter. *Fluency and Fluency Disorders*, 14–17.

Schum, R. (1986). *Counseling in speech and hearing practice*. Rockville, MD: National Student Speech-Language-Hearing Association.

Smart, J. (2001). *Disability, society, and the individual*. Gaithersburg, MD: Aspen.

Tetnowski, J. (2003, December). Demystifying our roles as counselors with adults who stutter. *Fluency and Fluency Disorders*, 7–10.

U. S. Department of Health and Human Services. (2003). *Summary of the HIPPA Rule*. Retrieved September 7, 2007, from http://www.hhs.gov/ocr/privacy summary.pdf

Walter, J., & Peller, J. (1992). *Becoming solution-focused in therapy*. New York: Brunner/Mazel.

Wisconsin Department of Public Instruction. (2004). *Student records and confidentiality*. Madison, WI: Author.

Chapter 9

ORAL LANGUAGE CURRICULUM STANDARDS INVENTORY (OL-CSI): AN AUTHENTIC ASSESSMENT APPROACH FOR SCHOOL-BASED SPEECH-LANGUAGE PATHOLOGISTS

RELATED VOCABULARY

authentic assessment   Assessment of performance while the student is engaged in a realistic learning context.

curriculum standard   A description of the achievement a student is expected to gain at a specific point in the scope and sequence of the school's curriculum.

deficit-driven   Describing an educational approach in which the focus is placed on a problem or weakness.

educationally relevant   Referring to content pertaining to the knowledge, skills, and attitudes that the student is learning in his or her curriculum.

Overview

As described in Chapter One, school-based speech-language services grew out of a medical model that advocated for students to be "cured" of their delays, disorders, and differences by receiving "speech correction" lessons from a specially trained educator. The **deficit-driven** attitudes of the medical model shaped school-based services until the "Quiet Revolution" began to unfold in 1975. Thirty-odd years later, some school districts continue to operate from that somewhat archaic deficit-driven model. Perrone (1991) pointed out the pitfalls of typical assessment techniques, which provide an artificial, decontextualized view of the learner. Perrone's concerns have been echoed by the American Speech-Language-Hearing Association (ASHA, 2000): "Standard assessment protocols have not necessarily reflected the changes sought in the educational setting, but rather have tended to measure only the change in the specified deficit area" (p. 5).

The mandates for providing a free and appropriate public education in the least restrictive environment have chipped away at the deficit-driven attitudes as recently as the reauthorization of the Individuals with Disabilities Education Improvement Act (IDEA) of 2004. Today's school-based speech-language pathologists (SLPs) must collaborate with other educators and design **educationally relevant** individualized education programs (IEPs) that are curriculum-based and more responsive to educational contexts.

The logical link between more educationally relevant IEPs and more educationally relevant assessment tools is becoming clearer. As stated by the ASHA (2000), "It will no longer be appropriate to provide, as some IEPs have done in the past, test scores as sole examples of performance levels" (p. 9).

School-based SLPs are exploring the use of **authentic assessment** tools as they meet the challenge of assessing a student's strengths, needs, interests, and learning styles in educational contexts. An authentic assessment approach to diagnostic processes has a solid research base behind it (Campbell, 2000; Choate & Evans, 1992; Diez & Moon, 1992; Lund & Duchan, 1993; Meyer, 1992; Schraeder, Quinn, Stockman & Miller, 1999; Thompson, 2001; Udvari-Solner & Thousand, 1995). The Oral Language Curriculum Standards Inventory (OL-CSI), presented as Appendix 9–1 at the end of this chapter, is an authentic assessment approach, incorporating a clearly stated **curriculum standard** for each grade level, that focuses on the student's oral language skills in the educational environment. The performance indicators have been synthesized from model academic oral language content standards published by educational agencies across the United States (Virginia Department of Education, 2005; Palo Alto Unified School District, 2005; Ohio Statewide Language Task Force, 1990; Tennessee Department of Education, 2005; Wisconsin Department of Public Instruction, 2005; Wisconsin Model Early Learning Standards, 2005a, 2005b).

The SLP is encouraged to use at least three different sources of information when completing the OL-CSI. Some examples are a classroom observation, a parent interview, and a peer-to-peer interaction in an unstructured setting such as the school playground. If the student is mature enough to do a self-assessment, this also may be a source of information. As documented by Goodrich (1996) and Goodrich Andrade (2000), involving the student, if developmentally capable, in a self-reflective process may have the effect of ultimately increasing the student's learning on IEP goals.

References

American Speech-Language-Hearing Association. (2000). *Developing educationally relevant IEPs: A technical assistance document for speech-language pathologists.* Reston, VA: Council for Exceptional Children.

Campbell, D. (2000, January). Authentic assessment and authentic standards. *Phi Delta Kappan, 81*(5), 405–407.

Choate, J. S, & Evans, S. (1992). Authentic assessment of special learners: Problem or promise? *Preventing School Failure, 37*(1), 6–9.

Diez, M., & Moon, J. (1992). What do we want students to know? . . . And other important questions. *Educational Leadership, 49*(8), 38–41.

Goodrich, H. (1996). *Student self-assessment: At the intersection of metacognition and authentic assessment.* Unpublished doctoral dissertation, Harvard University, Cambridge, MA.

Goodrich Andrade, H. (2000). Using rubrics to promote thinking and learning. *Educational Leadership, 57*(5), 13-18.

Lund, N., & Duchan, J. (1993). *Assessing children's language in naturalistic contexts.* Englewood Cliffs, NJ: Prentice-Hall.

Meyer, C. (1992). What's the difference between authentic and performance assessment? *Educational Leadership, 49*(8), 39-40.

Palo Alto Unified School District. (2005). *Speaking and listening skills.* Retrieved January 20, 2005, from http://pausd.org/parents/curriculum/elementary/first.shtml

Ohio Statewide Language Task Force. (1991). Developmental milestones: Language behaviors. In *Ohio handbook for the identification, evaluation and placement of children with language problems.* Columbus, OH: Ohio Department of Education.

Perrone, V. (1991). *Expanding student assessment.* Alexandria, VA: Association for Supervision and Curriculum Development.

Schraeder, T., Quinn, M., Stockman, I., & Miller, J. (1999). Authentic assessment as an approach to preschool speech-language screening. *American Journal of Speech-Language Pathology, 8*, 195-200.

Tennessee Department of Education. (2005). *Oral language K-8 curriculum standards.* Retrieved January 20, 2005, from http://www.state.tn.us/education/ci/cistandards2001/la/cilagkaccomp.html

Thompson, S. (2001). The authentic standards movement and its evil twin. *Phi Delta Kappan, 82*(5), 358-362.

Udvari-Solner, A., & Thousand, J. (1995). Promising practices that foster inclusive education. In R. Villa & J. Thousand (Eds.), *Creating an inclusive school.* Alexandria, VA: Association for Supervision and Curriculum Development.

Virginia Department of Education. (2005). *Oral language K-12 curriculum standards.* Retrieved January 20, 2005, from http://www.pen.k12.va.us/VDOE/Superintendent/Sols/2002/English1.doc

Wisconsin Department of Public Instruction. (2005). *Oral Language K-12 curriculum standards.* Retrieved January, 20, 2005, from http://www.dpi.state.wi.us/standards/elac4.html

Wisconsin Model Early Learning Standards. (2005a). *Social and emotional development.* Retrieved January 20, 2005, from http://www.collaboratingpartners.com

Wisconsin Model Early Learning Standards. (2005b). *Speaking and communicating.* Retrieved January 20, 2005, from http://www.collaboratingpartners.com

APPENDIX 9–1

Oral Language Curriculum Standards Inventory (OL-CSI)

Directions for Administering the OL-CSI

Select at least three information sources. Possible information sources may include, but are not limited to, observation of a peer-to-peer interaction in an unstructured setting within the school (e.g., the lunchroom), observation in a community-based setting (e.g., day care), observation of a parent-child interaction, observation of a sibling interaction, information gained from a parent interview, information gained from a student's self-reflection, analysis of a video sample, analysis of an audio sample, classroom observation, teacher interview, and a physician's note.

Begin at the academic level that matches the student's chronological age. If 75% of performance indicators or more within that grade level are scored as 2 or 1 on the rating scale, move to the next lower grade level and continue the rating process. Continue working backwards until at least 75% of the performance indicators are rated within a 3 or 4. The student's functional oral language range is reflected by the grade level at which at least 75% of the performance indicators are rated as 3 or 4.

The OL-CSI is an informal assessment tool, and no psychometric measures should be applied. The OL-CSI should not be the only assessment instrument used for evaluation purposes, nor should it be considered a formal assessment tool with psychometric scales. It should be used as part of the full repertoire of formal and informal tools used to collect assessment data.

The OL-CSI uses a five-point rating scale, as follows:

0 = *not assessed*

1 = *below expected benchmark performance* (the student cannot make adequate yearly progress with this level of performance)

2 = *inconsistent performance* (the student does not demonstrate adequate performance in at least three out of five consecutive school days)

3 = *adequate performance* (the student can make adequate yearly progress with this level of performance)

4 = *strength* (the student shows confidence and appears to be making adequate yearly progress)

Preschool/Kindergarten Oral Language Skills

	0	1	2	3	4
Uses 3- to 5-word utterances	☐	☐	☐	☐	☐
Responds to questions 75% of the time	☐	☐	☐	☐	☐
Produces *m,* h, w, p, b, d, f, k, g, n, j, t, th, within conventions of Standard American English or a recognized dialect	☐	☐	☐	☐	☐
Produces tk, kw, pl, bl, kl, gl, and fl within conventions of Standard American English or a recognized dialect	☐	☐	☐	☐	☐
10% or fewer utterances contain mazes	☐	☐	☐	☐	☐
Speaks at a rate approximately 39 words per minute	☐	☐	☐	☐	☐
Uses negatives (no, not, don't, can't)	☐	☐	☐	☐	☐
Uses verb inflections within conventions of Standard American English or a recognized dialect	☐	☐	☐	☐	☐
Uses plurals within the conventions of Standard American English or a recognized dialect	☐	☐	☐	☐	☐
Uses correct word order in sentences	☐	☐	☐	☐	☐
Uses adjectives	☐	☐	☐	☐	☐
Initiates communication with others	☐	☐	☐	☐	☐
Requests clarification	☐	☐	☐	☐	☐
Gives clarification	☐	☐	☐	☐	☐
Answers *who*, *what*, *where*, and *when* questions	☐	☐	☐	☐	☐
Follows two-step directions	☐	☐	☐	☐	☐
Engages in conversation with turn taking	☐	☐	☐	☐	☐
Stays on topic for 3 to 5 minutes	☐	☐	☐	☐	☐
Verbally interacts with one or more children	☐	☐	☐	☐	☐
Seeks out peers as play partners	☐	☐	☐	☐	☐
Participates successfully as a member of a group	☐	☐	☐	☐	☐
Uses words to resolve conflicts	☐	☐	☐	☐	☐
Forms explanations based on trial and error, observations, and explorations	☐	☐	☐	☐	☐

First Grade Oral Language Skills

	0	1	2	3	4
Uses 5- to 7-word utterances	☐	☐	☐	☐	☐
Responds to questions 80% of the time	☐	☐	☐	☐	☐
Produces m, h, w, p, b, d, f, k, g, n, j, t, th, l, f, v, sh, ch, th, and j within conventions of Standard American English or a recognized dialect	☐	☐	☐	☐	☐
Produces tk, kw, pl, bl, kl, gl, fl, or, gr, br,tr, dr kr, gr, and fr within conventions of Standard American English or a recognized dialect	☐	☐	☐	☐	☐
10% or fewer utterances contain mazes	☐	☐	☐	☐	☐
Speaks at a rate approximately 84 words per minute	☐	☐	☐	☐	☐
Uses negatives (no, not, don't, can't)	☐	☐	☐	☐	☐
Uses conjunctions	☐	☐	☐	☐	☐
Uses personal pronouns	☐	☐	☐	☐	☐
Uses verb inflections within conventions of Standard American English or a recognized dialect	☐	☐	☐	☐	☐
Uses plurals within the conventions of Standard American English or a recognized dialect	☐	☐	☐	☐	☐
Retells a story using a *first*, *next*, *then*, and *last* sequence	☐	☐	☐	☐	☐
Recites short poems, rhymes, and songs in choral response settings	☐	☐	☐	☐	☐
Defines objects by use	☐	☐	☐	☐	☐
Uses correct word order in sentences	☐	☐	☐	☐	☐
Uses adjectives	☐	☐	☐	☐	☐
Initiates communication with others	☐	☐	☐	☐	☐
Requests clarification	☐	☐	☐	☐	☐
Gives clarification	☐	☐	☐	☐	☐
Answers *who*, *what*, *where*, *when*, *why*, and *how* questions	☐	☐	☐	☐	☐
Follows two-step directions	☐	☐	☐	☐	☐
Engages in conversation with turn taking	☐	☐	☐	☐	☐
Can adapt or change conversation to fit the circumstance	☐	☐	☐	☐	☐
Stays on topic for 7 to 12 minutes	☐	☐	☐	☐	☐
Adds or deletes sounds to make new words	☐	☐	☐	☐	☐
Counts syllables in 3-syllable words	☐	☐	☐	☐	☐
Gives opposites	☐	☐	☐	☐	☐
Creates a rhyme	☐	☐	☐	☐	☐
Blends sounds to make word parts and words with 1 to 3 syllables	☐	☐	☐	☐	☐

Second Grade Oral Language Skills

	0	1	2	3	4
Uses 5- to 7-word utterances	☐	☐	☐	☐	☐
Responds to questions 80% of the time	☐	☐	☐	☐	☐
Produces m, h, w, p, b, d, f, k, g, n, j, t, th, l, f, v, sh, ch, th, j, r, s, and z within conventions of Standard American English or a recognized dialect	☐	☐	☐	☐	☐
Produces tk, kw, pl, bl, kl, gl, fl, pr, gr, br, tr, dr, kr, gr, fr, sp, st, sk, sm, sn, sw, sl, skw, spl, spr, str, skr, and thr within conventions of Standard American English or a recognized dialect	☐	☐	☐	☐	☐
10% or fewer utterances contain mazes	☐	☐	☐	☐	☐
Speaks at a rate approximately 84 words per minute	☐	☐	☐	☐	☐
Uses negatives (no, not, don't, can't)	☐	☐	☐	☐	☐
Uses conjunctions	☐	☐	☐	☐	☐
Uses personal pronouns	☐	☐	☐	☐	☐
Uses verb inflections within conventions of Standard American English or a recognized dialect	☐	☐	☐	☐	☐
Uses plurals within the conventions of Standard American English or a recognized dialect	☐	☐	☐	☐	☐
Creates a story to share with others	☐	☐	☐	☐	☐
Summarizes information presented orally by others	☐	☐	☐	☐	☐
Creates and participate in oral dramatic activities	☐	☐	☐	☐	☐
Recites short poems, rhymes, and songs in choral response settings	☐	☐	☐	☐	☐
Defines objects by use	☐	☐	☐	☐	☐
Uses correct word order in sentences	☐	☐	☐	☐	☐
Uses adjectives	☐	☐	☐	☐	☐
Initiates communication with others	☐	☐	☐	☐	☐
Requests clarification	☐	☐	☐	☐	☐
Gives clarification	☐	☐	☐	☐	☐
Answers *who*, *what*, *where*, *when*, *why*, and *how* questions	☐	☐	☐	☐	☐
Gives three- and four-step directions	☐	☐	☐	☐	☐
Engages in conversation with turn taking	☐	☐	☐	☐	☐
Adapts or changes conversation to fit the circumstance	☐	☐	☐	☐	☐
Uses oral language to persuade	☐	☐	☐	☐	☐
Uses oral language to entertain	☐	☐	☐	☐	☐
Narrates a personal story	☐	☐	☐	☐	☐

Second Grade Oral Language Skills *(continued)*	0	1	2	3	4
Stays on topic for 7 to 12 minutes	☐	☐	☐	☐	☐
Adds or deletes sounds to make new words	☐	☐	☐	☐	☐
Counts syllables in 3-syllable words	☐	☐	☐	☐	☐
Gives synonyms and antonyms	☐	☐	☐	☐	☐
Creates a rhyme	☐	☐	☐	☐	☐
Blends sounds to make word parts and words with 1 to 3 syllables	☐	☐	☐	☐	☐

Third Grade Oral Language Skills	0	1	2	3	4
Uses 7- to 8-word utterances	☐	☐	☐	☐	☐
Responds to questions 80% of the time					
Produces m, h, w, p, b, d, f, k, g, n, j, t, th, l, f, v, sh, ch, th, j, r, s, and z within conventions of Standard American English or a recognized dialect	☐	☐	☐	☐	☐
Produces tk, kw, pl, bl, kl, gl, fl, pr, gr, br, tr, dr, kr, gr, fr, sp, st, sk, sm, sn, sw, sl, skw, spl, spr, str, skr, and thr within conventions of Standard American English or a recognized dialect	☐	☐	☐	☐	☐
8% or fewer utterances contain mazes	☐	☐	☐	☐	☐
Speaks at a rate approximately 97 words per minute	☐	☐	☐	☐	☐
Uses negatives (no, not, don't, can't)	☐	☐	☐	☐	☐
Uses conjunctions	☐	☐	☐	☐	☐
Uses personal pronouns	☐	☐	☐	☐	☐
Uses verb inflections within conventions of Standard American English or a recognized dialect	☐	☐	☐	☐	☐
Uses plurals within the conventions of Standard American English or a recognized dialect	☐	☐	☐	☐	☐
Creates a story to share with others	☐	☐	☐	☐	☐
Summarizes information presented orally by others	☐	☐	☐	☐	☐
Creates and participate in oral dramatic activities	☐	☐	☐	☐	☐
Recites short poems, rhymes, and songs in choral response settings	☐	☐	☐	☐	☐
Defines objects by size, shape, function, and location	☐	☐	☐	☐	☐
Uses correct word order in sentences	☐	☐	☐	☐	☐
Uses adjectives	☐	☐	☐	☐	☐
Initiates communication with others	☐	☐	☐	☐	☐
Requests clarification	☐	☐	☐	☐	☐
Gives clarification	☐	☐	☐	☐	☐

Third Grade Oral Language Skills *(continued)*

	0	1	2	3	4
Answers *who, what, where, when, why,* and *how* questions	☐	☐	☐	☐	☐
Gives three- and four-step directions	☐	☐	☐	☐	☐
Engages in conversation with turn taking	☐	☐	☐	☐	☐
Adapts or changes conversation to fit the circumstance	☐	☐	☐	☐	☐
Uses oral language to persuade	☐	☐	☐	☐	☐
Uses oral language to entertain; uses humor	☐	☐	☐	☐	☐
Narrates a personal story	☐	☐	☐	☐	☐
Stays on topic for 7 to 12 minutes	☐	☐	☐	☐	☐
Adds or deletes sounds to make new words	☐	☐	☐	☐	☐
Counts syllables in 3-syllable words	☐	☐	☐	☐	☐
Gives synonyms and antonyms	☐	☐	☐	☐	☐
Creates a rhyme	☐	☐	☐	☐	☐
Blends sounds to make word parts and words with 1 to 3 syllables	☐	☐	☐	☐	☐
Gives a brief oral report in front of a group	☐	☐	☐	☐	☐
Uses the telephone and takes messages	☐	☐	☐	☐	☐

Fourth Grade Oral Language Skills

	0	1	2	3	4
Uses 8- to 9-word utterances	☐	☐	☐	☐	☐
Responds to questions 85% of the time	☐	☐	☐	☐	☐
Produces m, h, w, p, b, d, f, k, g, n, j, t, th, l, f, v, sh, ch, th, j, r, s, and z within conventions of Standard American English or a recognized dialect	☐	☐	☐	☐	☐
Produces tk, kw, pl, bl, kl, gl, fl, pr, gr, br, tr, dr, kr, gr, fr, sp, st, sk, sm, sn, sw, sl, skw, spl, spr, str, skr, and thr within conventions of Standard American English or a recognized dialect	☐	☐	☐	☐	☐
8% or fewer utterances contain mazes	☐	☐	☐	☐	☐
Speaks at a rate approximately 130 words per minute	☐	☐	☐	☐	☐
Uses negatives (no, not, don't, can't)	☐	☐	☐	☐	☐
Uses conjunctions	☐	☐	☐	☐	☐
Uses personal pronouns	☐	☐	☐	☐	☐
Uses verb inflections within conventions of Standard American English or a recognized dialect	☐	☐	☐	☐	☐
Uses plurals within the conventions of Standard American English or a recognized dialect	☐	☐	☐	☐	☐
Creates a story to share with others	☐	☐	☐	☐	☐

Fourth Grade Oral Language Skills *(continued)*

	0	1	2	3	4
Summarizes information presented orally by others	☐	☐	☐	☐	☐
Participates in group oral, choral, shadow, or echo readings	☐	☐	☐	☐	☐
Recites short poems, rhymes, and songs	☐	☐	☐	☐	☐
Defines objects by size, shape, function, and location	☐	☐	☐	☐	☐
Uses correct word order in sentences	☐	☐	☐	☐	☐
Uses eight parts of speech (noun, pronoun, verb, adverb, conjunction, and so on)	☐	☐	☐	☐	☐
Initiates communication with others	☐	☐	☐	☐	☐
Requests clarification	☐	☐	☐	☐	☐
Gives clarification	☐	☐	☐	☐	☐
Answers *who, what, where, when, why,* and *how* questions	☐	☐	☐	☐	☐
Gives directions for games	☐	☐	☐	☐	☐
Engages in conversation with turn taking	☐	☐	☐	☐	☐
Adapts or changes conversation to fit the circumstance	☐	☐	☐	☐	☐
Uses oral language to persuade	☐	☐	☐	☐	☐
Uses oral language to entertain	☐	☐	☐	☐	☐
Presents autobiographical or fictional stories that recount events effectively to large or small audiences	☐	☐	☐	☐	☐
Stays on topic for 20 to 30 minutes	☐	☐	☐	☐	☐
Adds or deletes sounds to make new words	☐	☐	☐	☐	☐
Counts syllables in 3-syllable words	☐	☐	☐	☐	☐
Creates a rhyme	☐	☐	☐	☐	☐
Blends sounds to make word parts and words with 1 to 4 syllables	☐	☐	☐	☐	☐
Speaks from notes or a brief outline, communicates precise information	☐	☐	☐	☐	☐
Uses the telephone and takes messages	☐	☐	☐	☐	☐
Uses verbal humor	☐	☐	☐	☐	☐
Reads aloud from previously read material	☐	☐	☐	☐	☐
Distinguishes between fact and fiction and provides evidence	☐	☐	☐	☐	☐
Distinguishes between fact and opinion and provides evidence	☐	☐	☐	☐	☐
Uses a graphic organizer for verbal presentations	☐	☐	☐	☐	☐
Predicts outcomes	☐	☐	☐	☐	☐
Draws conclusions	☐	☐	☐	☐	☐
Uses prefixes, suffices, homonyms, synonyms, antonyms, and word analogies	☐	☐	☐	☐	☐
Uses cause and effect	☐	☐	☐	☐	☐

Fifth Grade Oral Language Skills

	0	1	2	3	4
Uses 9- to 10-word utterances	☐	☐	☐	☐	☐
Responds to questions 85% of the time	☐	☐	☐	☐	☐
Produces m, h, w, p, b, d, f, k, g, n, j, t, th, l, f, v, sh, ch, th, j, r, s, and z within conventions of Standard American English or a recognized dialect	☐	☐	☐	☐	☐
Produces tk, kw, pl, bl, kl, gl, fl, pr, gr, br, tr, dr, kr, gr, fr, sp, st, sk, sm, sn, sw, sl, skw, spl, spr, str, skr, and thr within conventions of Standard American English or a recognized dialect	☐	☐	☐	☐	☐
8% or fewer utterances contain mazes	☐	☐	☐	☐	☐
Speaks at a rate approximately 128 words per minute	☐	☐	☐	☐	☐
Uses negatives (no, not, don't, can't)	☐	☐	☐	☐	☐
Uses conjunctions	☐	☐	☐	☐	☐
Uses personal pronouns	☐	☐	☐	☐	☐
Uses verb inflections within conventions of Standard American English or a recognized dialect	☐	☐	☐	☐	☐
Uses plurals within the conventions of Standard American English or a recognized dialect	☐	☐	☐	☐	☐
Creates a story to share with others	☐	☐	☐	☐	☐
Summarizes information presented orally by others	☐	☐	☐	☐	☐
Participates in group oral, choral, shadow, or echo readings	☐	☐	☐	☐	☐
Recites short poems, rhymes, and songs	☐	☐	☐	☐	☐
Defines objects by size, shape, material makeup, function, location	☐	☐	☐	☐	☐
Uses correct word order in sentences	☐	☐	☐	☐	☐
Uses eight parts of speech (noun, pronoun, verb, adverb, conjunction, and so on)	☐	☐	☐	☐	☐
Initiates communication with others	☐	☐	☐	☐	☐
Requests clarification	☐	☐	☐	☐	☐
Gives clarification	☐	☐	☐	☐	☐
Answers *who*, *what*, *where*, *when*, *why*, and *how* questions	☐	☐	☐	☐	☐
Gives directions for games	☐	☐	☐	☐	☐
Engages in conversation with turn taking	☐	☐	☐	☐	☐
Adapts or changes conversation to fit the circumstance	☐	☐	☐	☐	☐
Uses oral language to persuade	☐	☐	☐	☐	☐
Uses oral language to entertain	☐	☐	☐	☐	☐

Fifth Grade Oral Language Skills *(continued)*

	0	1	2	3	4
Presents autobiographical or fictional stories that recount events effectively to large or small audiences	☐	☐	☐	☐	☐
Stays on topic for 20 to 30 minutes	☐	☐	☐	☐	☐
Adds or deletes sounds to make new words	☐	☐	☐	☐	☐
Counts syllables in 3- to 5-syllable words	☐	☐	☐	☐	☐
Creates a rhyme	☐	☐	☐	☐	☐
Blends sounds to make word parts and words with 1 to 5 syllables	☐	☐	☐	☐	☐
Speaks from notes or a brief outline, communicates precise information	☐	☐	☐	☐	☐
Uses the telephone and takes messages	☐	☐	☐	☐	☐
Uses verbal humor	☐	☐	☐	☐	☐
Reads aloud from previously read material	☐	☐	☐	☐	☐
Distinguishes between fact and fiction and provides evidence	☐	☐	☐	☐	☐
Distinguishes between fact and opinion and provides evidence	☐	☐	☐	☐	☐
Uses a graphic organizer for verbal presentations	☐	☐	☐	☐	☐
Uses visual aids to support a verbal presentation	☐	☐	☐	☐	☐
Predicts outcomes	☐	☐	☐	☐	☐
Draws conclusions and shares responses in group learning activities	☐	☐	☐	☐	☐
Summarizes information gathered in group activities	☐	☐	☐	☐	☐
Uses prefixes, suffices, homonyms, synonyms, antonyms, and word analogies	☐	☐	☐	☐	☐
Uses cause and effect	☐	☐	☐	☐	☐

Sixth Grade Oral Language Skills

	0	1	2	3	4
Uses 9- to 10-word utterances	☐	☐	☐	☐	☐
Responds to questions 85% of the time	☐	☐	☐	☐	☐
Produces m, h, w, p, b, d, f, k, g, n, j, t, th, l, f, v, sh, ch, th, j, r, s, and z within conventions of Standard American English or a recognized dialect	☐	☐	☐	☐	☐
Produces tk, kw, pl, bl, kl, gl, fl, pr, gr, br, tr, dr, kr, gr, fr, sp, st, sk, sm, sn, sw, sl, skw, spl, spr, str, skr, and thr within conventions of Standard American English or a recognized dialect	☐	☐	☐	☐	☐
8% or fewer utterances contain mazes	☐	☐	☐	☐	☐
Speaks at a rate approximately 128 words per minute	☐	☐	☐	☐	☐
Uses negatives (no, not, don't, can't)	☐	☐	☐	☐	☐

Sixth Grade Oral Language Skills *(continued)*

	0	1	2	3	4
Uses conjunctions	☐	☐	☐	☐	☐
Uses personal pronouns	☐	☐	☐	☐	☐
Uses verb inflections within conventions of Standard American English or a recognized dialect	☐	☐	☐	☐	☐
Uses plurals within the conventions of Standard American English or a recognized dialect	☐	☐	☐	☐	☐
Creates a story to share with others	☐	☐	☐	☐	☐
Summarizes information presented orally by others	☐	☐	☐	☐	☐
Participates in group oral, choral, shadow, or echo readings	☐	☐	☐	☐	☐
Recites short poems, rhymes, and songs	☐	☐	☐	☐	☐
Defines objects by size, shape, material makeup, function, location	☐	☐	☐	☐	☐
Uses correct word order in sentences	☐	☐	☐	☐	☐
Uses eight parts of speech (noun, pronoun, verb, adverb, conjunction, and so on)	☐	☐	☐	☐	☐
Initiates communication with others	☐	☐	☐	☐	☐
Requests clarification	☐	☐	☐	☐	☐
Gives clarification	☐	☐	☐	☐	☐
Answers *who*, *what*, *where*, *when*, *why*, and *how* questions	☐	☐	☐	☐	☐
Gives directions for games	☐	☐	☐	☐	☐
Engages in conversation with turn taking	☐	☐	☐	☐	☐
Adapts or changes conversation to fit the circumstance	☐	☐	☐	☐	☐
Uses oral language to persuade	☐	☐	☐	☐	☐
Uses oral language to entertain	☐	☐	☐	☐	☐
Presents autobiographical or fictional stories that recount events effectively to large or small audiences	☐	☐	☐	☐	☐
Stays on topic for 20 to 30 minutes	☐	☐	☐	☐	☐
Adds or deletes sounds to make new words	☐	☐	☐	☐	☐
Counts syllables in 3- to 5-syllable words	☐	☐	☐	☐	☐
Creates a rhyme	☐	☐	☐	☐	☐
Blends sounds to make word parts and words with 1 to 5 syllables	☐	☐	☐	☐	☐
Speaks from notes or a brief outline, communicates precise information	☐	☐	☐	☐	☐
Uses the telephone and takes messages	☐	☐	☐	☐	☐
Uses verbal humor	☐	☐	☐	☐	☐

Sixth Grade Oral Language Skills *(continued)*

	0	1	2	3	4
Reads aloud from previously read material	☐	☐	☐	☐	☐
Distinguishes between fact and fiction and provides evidence	☐	☐	☐	☐	☐
Distinguishes between fact and opinion and provides evidence	☐	☐	☐	☐	☐
Uses a graphic organizer for verbal presentations	☐	☐	☐	☐	☐
Uses visual aids to support a verbal presentation	☐	☐	☐	☐	☐
Predicts outcomes	☐	☐	☐	☐	☐
Draws conclusions and shares responses in group learning activities	☐	☐	☐	☐	☐
Summarizes information gathered in group activities	☐	☐	☐	☐	☐
Uses prefixes, suffices, homonyms, synonyms, antonyms, and word analogies	☐	☐	☐	☐	☐
Uses cause and effect	☐	☐	☐	☐	☐
Evaluates own contributions to discussions	☐	☐	☐	☐	☐
Analyzes the effectiveness of participant interactions	☐	☐	☐	☐	☐
Compares and contrasts differing viewpoints	☐	☐	☐	☐	☐

Seventh Grade Oral Language Skills

	0	1	2	3	4
Uses 9- to 10-word utterances	☐	☐	☐	☐	☐
Responds to questions 85% of the time	☐	☐	☐	☐	☐
Produces m, h, w, p, b, d, f, k, g, n, j, t, th, l, f, v, sh, ch, th, j, r, s, and z within conventions of Standard American English or a recognized dialect	☐	☐	☐	☐	☐
Produces tk, kw, pl, bl, kl, gl, fl, pr, gr, br, tr, dr, kr, gr, fr, sp, st, sk, sm, sn, sw, sl, skw, spl, spr, str, skr, and thr within conventions of Standard American English or a recognized dialect	☐	☐	☐	☐	☐
8% or fewer utterances contain mazes	☐	☐	☐	☐	☐
Speaks at a rate approximately 128 words per minute	☐	☐	☐	☐	☐
Uses negatives (no, not, don't, can't)	☐	☐	☐	☐	☐
Uses conjunctions	☐	☐	☐	☐	☐
Uses personal pronouns	☐	☐	☐	☐	☐
Uses verb inflections within conventions of Standard American English or a recognized dialect	☐	☐	☐	☐	☐
Uses plurals within the conventions of Standard American English or a recognized dialect	☐	☐	☐	☐	☐
Creates a story to share with others	☐	☐	☐	☐	☐
Summarizes information presented orally by others	☐	☐	☐	☐	☐

Seventh Grade Oral Language Skills *(continued)*

	0	1	2	3	4
Participates in group oral, choral, shadow, or echo readings	☐	☐	☐	☐	☐
Recites short poems, rhymes, and songs	☐	☐	☐	☐	☐
Defines objects by size, shape, material makeup, function, location	☐	☐	☐	☐	☐
Uses correct word order in sentences	☐	☐	☐	☐	☐
Uses eight parts of speech (noun, pronoun, verb, adverb, conjunction, and so on)	☐	☐	☐	☐	☐
Initiates communication with others	☐	☐	☐	☐	☐
Requests clarification	☐	☐	☐	☐	☐
Gives clarification	☐	☐	☐	☐	☐
Answers *who*, *what*, *where*, *when*, *why*, and *how* questions	☐	☐	☐	☐	☐
Gives directions for games	☐	☐	☐	☐	☐
Engages in conversation with turn taking	☐	☐	☐	☐	☐
Adapts or changes conversation to fit the circumstance	☐	☐	☐	☐	☐
Uses oral language to persuade	☐	☐	☐	☐	☐
Uses oral language to entertain	☐	☐	☐	☐	☐
Presents autobiographical or fictional stories that recount events effectively to large or small audiences	☐	☐	☐	☐	☐
Stays on topic for 20 to 30 minutes	☐	☐	☐	☐	☐
Adds or deletes sounds to make new words	☐	☐	☐	☐	☐
Counts syllables in 3- to 5-syllable words	☐	☐	☐	☐	☐
Creates a rhyme	☐	☐	☐	☐	☐
Blends sounds to make word parts and words with 1 to 5 syllables	☐	☐	☐	☐	☐
Speaks from notes or a brief outline, communicates precise information	☐	☐	☐	☐	☐
Uses the telephone and takes messages	☐	☐	☐	☐	☐
Uses verbal humor	☐	☐	☐	☐	☐
Reads aloud from previously read material	☐	☐	☐	☐	☐
Distinguishes between fact and fiction and provides evidence	☐	☐	☐	☐	☐
Distinguishes between fact and opinion and provides evidence	☐	☐	☐	☐	☐
Uses a graphic organizer for verbal presentations	☐	☐	☐	☐	☐
Uses visual aids to support a verbal presentation	☐	☐	☐	☐	☐
Predicts outcomes	☐	☐	☐	☐	☐
Draws conclusions and shares responses in group learning activities	☐	☐	☐	☐	☐

Seventh Grade Oral Language Skills (continued)	0	1	2	3	4
Summarizes information gathered in group activities	☐	☐	☐	☐	☐
Uses prefixes, suffices, homonyms, synonyms, antonyms, and word analogies	☐	☐	☐	☐	☐
Uses cause and effect	☐	☐	☐	☐	☐
Evaluates self-contributions to discussions	☐	☐	☐	☐	☐
Analyzes the effectiveness of participant interactions	☐	☐	☐	☐	☐
Compares and contrasts differing viewpoints	☐	☐	☐	☐	☐
Compares and contrasts verbal and nonverbal messages	☐	☐	☐	☐	☐
Describes persuasive messages from nonprint media (TV, radio, and video)	☐	☐	☐	☐	☐
Describes how word choice conveys viewpoint	☐	☐	☐	☐	☐

Eighth Grade Oral Language Skills	0	1	2	3	4
Uses 9- to 11-word utterances	☐	☐	☐	☐	☐
Responds to questions 85% of the time	☐	☐	☐	☐	☐
Produces m, h, w, p, b, d, f, k, g, n, j, t, th, l, f, v, sh, ch, th, j, r, s, and z within conventions of Standard American English or a recognized dialect	☐	☐	☐	☐	☐
Produces tk, kw, pl, bl, kl, gl, fl, pr, gr, br, tr, dr, kr, gr, fr, sp, st, sk, sm, sn, sw, sl, skw, spl, spr, str, skr, and thr within conventions of Standard American English or a recognized dialect	☐	☐	☐	☐	☐
8% or fewer utterances contain mazes	☐	☐	☐	☐	☐
Speaks at a rate approximately 143 words per minute	☐	☐	☐	☐	☐
Uses negatives (no, not, don't, can't)	☐	☐	☐	☐	☐
Uses conjunctions	☐	☐	☐	☐	☐
Uses personal pronouns	☐	☐	☐	☐	☐
Uses verb inflections within conventions of Standard American English or a recognized dialect	☐	☐	☐	☐	☐
Uses plurals within the conventions of Standard American English or a recognized dialect	☐	☐	☐	☐	☐
Creates a story to share with others	☐	☐	☐	☐	☐
Summarizes information presented orally by others	☐	☐	☐	☐	☐
Participates in group oral, choral, shadow, or echo readings	☐	☐	☐	☐	☐
Performs expressive oral readings of prose, poetry, and drama	☐	☐	☐	☐	☐
Defines objects by size, shape, material makeup, function, location	☐	☐	☐	☐	☐
Uses correct word order in sentences	☐	☐	☐	☐	☐

Eighth Grade Oral Language Skills *(continued)*

	0	1	2	3	4
Uses eight parts of speech (noun, pronoun, verb, adverb, conjunction, and so on)	☐	☐	☐	☐	☐
Initiates communication with others	☐	☐	☐	☐	☐
Requests clarification	☐	☐	☐	☐	☐
Gives clarification	☐	☐	☐	☐	☐
Answers *who*, *what*, *where*, *when*, *why*, and *how* questions	☐	☐	☐	☐	☐
Gives directions for games	☐	☐	☐	☐	☐
Engages in conversation with turn taking	☐	☐	☐	☐	☐
Adapts or changes conversation to fit the circumstance	☐	☐	☐	☐	☐
Uses oral language to persuade	☐	☐	☐	☐	☐
Uses oral language to entertain	☐	☐	☐	☐	☐
Presents autobiographical or fictional stories that recount events effectively to large or small audiences	☐	☐	☐	☐	☐
Stays on topic for 20 to 30 minutes	☐	☐	☐	☐	☐
Adds or deletes sounds to make new words	☐	☐	☐	☐	☐
Counts syllables in 3- to 5-syllable words	☐	☐	☐	☐	☐
Creates a rhyme	☐	☐	☐	☐	☐
Blends sounds to make word parts and words with 1 to 5 syllables	☐	☐	☐	☐	☐
Speaks from notes or a brief outline, communicates precise information	☐	☐	☐	☐	☐
Uses the telephone and takes messages	☐	☐	☐	☐	☐
Uses verbal humor	☐	☐	☐	☐	☐
Reads aloud from previously read material	☐	☐	☐	☐	☐
Distinguishes between fact and fiction and provides evidence	☐	☐	☐	☐	☐
Distinguishes between fact and opinion and provides evidence	☐	☐	☐	☐	☐
Speaking from notes or an outline, relates an experience in descriptive detail, with a sense of timing and decorum appropriate to the occasion	☐	☐	☐	☐	☐
Uses visual aids to support a verbal presentation	☐	☐	☐	☐	☐
Predicts outcomes	☐	☐	☐	☐	☐
Draws conclusions and shares responses in group learning activities	☐	☐	☐	☐	☐
Summarizes information gathered in group activities	☐	☐	☐	☐	☐
Uses prefixes, suffices, homonyms, synonyms, antonyms, and word analogies	☐	☐	☐	☐	☐

Eighth Grade Oral Language Skills *(continued)*

	0	1	2	3	4
Uses cause and effect	☐	☐	☐	☐	☐
Evaluates self-contributions to discussions	☐	☐	☐	☐	☐
Analyzes the effectiveness of participant interactions	☐	☐	☐	☐	☐
Compares and contrasts differing viewpoints	☐	☐	☐	☐	☐
Compares and contrasts verbal and nonverbal messages	☐	☐	☐	☐	☐
Describes persuasive messages from nonprint media (TV, radio, and video)	☐	☐	☐	☐	☐
Describes how word choice conveys viewpoint	☐	☐	☐	☐	☐
Shares brief impromptu remarks about topics of interest to self and others	☐	☐	☐	☐	☐
Conducts an interview	☐	☐	☐	☐	☐
Presents a coherent, comprehensive report on differing viewpoints on an issue, evaluating the content of the material presented, and organizing the presentation in a manner appropriate to the audience	☐	☐	☐	☐	☐
Differentiates between formal and informal contexts and employs an appropriate style of speaking, adjusting language, gestures, rate, and volume according to the audience and purpose	☐	☐	☐	☐	☐
Summarizes and explains information conveyed in an oral communication, accounting for the key ideas, structure, and relationship of parts to the whole	☐	☐	☐	☐	☐
Evaluates the reliability of information in a communication, using criteria based on prior knowledge of the speaker, the topic, and the context and on analysis of logic, evidence, propaganda devices, and language	☐	☐	☐	☐	☐
Explains and advances opinions by citing evidence and referring to sources	☐	☐	☐	☐	☐
Summarizes the main points of a discussion, orally and in writing, specifying areas of agreement and disagreement and paraphrasing contributions	☐	☐	☐	☐	☐
Displays and maintains facial expressions, body language, and other response cues that indicate respect for the speaker and attention to the discussion	☐	☐	☐	☐	☐
Participates in a discussion without dominating	☐	☐	☐	☐	☐
Distinguishes between supported and unsupported statements	☐	☐	☐	☐	☐
Describes the role of communication in everyday situations (e.g., advertising, informal social, business, formal social)	☐	☐	☐	☐	☐
Can use persuasion, argumentation, and debate as essential oral skills	☐	☐	☐	☐	☐
Applies assessment criteria to self-evaluation of oral presentations	☐	☐	☐	☐	☐

Ninth to Twelfth Grade Oral Language Skills

	0	1	2	3	4
Uses 9- to 10-word utterances	☐	☐	☐	☐	☐
Responds to questions 85% of the time	☐	☐	☐	☐	☐
Produces m, h, w, p, b, d, f, k, g, n, j, t, th, l, f, v, sh, ch, th, j, r, s, and z within conventions of Standard American English or a recognized dialect	☐	☐	☐	☐	☐
Produces tk, kw, pl, bl, kl, gl, fl, pr, gr, br, tr, dr, kr, gr, fr, sp, st, sk, sm, sn, sw, sl, skw, spl, spr, str, skr, and thr within conventions of Standard American English or a recognized dialect	☐	☐	☐	☐	☐
8% or fewer utterances contain mazes	☐	☐	☐	☐	☐
Speaks at a rate approximately 128 words per minute	☐	☐	☐	☐	☐
Uses negatives (no, not, don't, can't)	☐	☐	☐	☐	☐
Uses conjunctions	☐	☐	☐	☐	☐
Uses personal pronouns	☐	☐	☐	☐	☐
Uses verb inflections within conventions of Standard American English or a recognized dialect	☐	☐	☐	☐	☐
Uses plurals within the conventions of Standard American English or a recognized dialect	☐	☐	☐	☐	☐
Creates a story to share with others	☐	☐	☐	☐	☐
Summarizes information presented orally by others	☐	☐	☐	☐	☐
Participates in group oral, choral, shadow, or echo readings	☐	☐	☐	☐	☐
Performs expressive oral readings of prose, poetry, and drama	☐	☐	☐	☐	☐
Defines objects by size, shape, material makeup, function, location	☐	☐	☐	☐	☐
Uses correct word order in sentences	☐	☐	☐	☐	☐
Uses eight parts of speech (noun, pronoun, verb, adverb, conjunction, and so on)	☐	☐	☐	☐	☐
Initiates communication with others	☐	☐	☐	☐	☐
Requests clarification	☐	☐	☐	☐	☐
Gives clarification	☐	☐	☐	☐	☐
Answers *who*, *what*, *where*, *when*, *why*, and *how* questions	☐	☐	☐	☐	☐
Gives directions for games	☐	☐	☐	☐	☐
Engages in conversation with turn taking	☐	☐	☐	☐	☐
Adapts or changes conversation to fit the circumstance	☐	☐	☐	☐	☐
Uses oral language to persuade	☐	☐	☐	☐	☐
Uses oral language to entertain	☐	☐	☐	☐	☐

Ninth to Twelfth Grade Oral Language Skills (*continued*)

	0	1	2	3	4
Presents autobiographical or fictional stories that recount events effectively to large or small audiences	☐	☐	☐	☐	☐
Stays on topic for 20 to 30 minutes	☐	☐	☐	☐	☐
Adds or deletes sounds to make new words	☐	☐	☐	☐	☐
Counts syllables in 3- to 5-syllable words	☐	☐	☐	☐	☐
Creates a rhyme	☐	☐	☐	☐	☐
Blends sounds to make word parts and words with 1 to 5 syllables	☐	☐	☐	☐	☐
Speaks from notes or a brief outline, communicates precise information	☐	☐	☐	☐	☐
Uses the telephone and takes messages	☐	☐	☐	☐	☐
Uses verbal humor	☐	☐	☐	☐	☐
Reads aloud from previously read material	☐	☐	☐	☐	☐
Distinguishes between fact and fiction and provides evidence	☐	☐	☐	☐	☐
Distinguishes between fact and opinion and provides evidence	☐	☐	☐	☐	☐
Speaking from notes or an outline, relates an experience in descriptive detail, with a sense of timing and decorum appropriate to the occasion	☐	☐	☐	☐	☐
Uses visual aids to support a verbal presentation	☐	☐	☐	☐	☐
Predicts outcomes	☐	☐	☐	☐	☐
Draws conclusions and shares responses in group learning activities	☐	☐	☐	☐	☐
Summarizes information gathered in group activities	☐	☐	☐	☐	☐
Uses prefixes, suffices, homonyms, synonyms, antonyms, and word analogies	☐	☐	☐	☐	☐
Uses cause and effect	☐	☐	☐	☐	☐
Evaluates own contributions to discussions	☐	☐	☐	☐	☐
Analyzes the effectiveness of participant interactions	☐	☐	☐	☐	☐
Compares and contrasts differing viewpoints	☐	☐	☐	☐	☐
Compares and contrasts verbal and nonverbal messages	☐	☐	☐	☐	☐
Describes persuasive messages from nonprint media (TV, radio, and video)	☐	☐	☐	☐	☐
Describes how word choice conveys viewpoint	☐	☐	☐	☐	☐
Shares brief impromptu remarks about topics of interest to oneself and others	☐	☐	☐	☐	☐
Conducts an interview	☐	☐	☐	☐	☐

Ninth to Twelfth Grade Oral Language Skills *(continued)*

	0	1	2	3	4
Presents a coherent, comprehensive report on differing viewpoints on an issue, evaluating the content of the material presented, and organizing the presentation in a manner appropriate to the audience	☐	☐	☐	☐	☐
Differentiates between formal and informal contexts and employs an appropriate style of speaking, adjusting language, gestures, rate, and volume according to the audience and purpose	☐	☐	☐	☐	☐
Summarizes and explains information conveyed in an oral communication, accounting for the key ideas, structure, and relationship of parts to the whole	☐	☐	☐	☐	☐
Evaluates the reliability of information in a communication, using criteria based on prior knowledge of the speaker, the topic, and the context and on analysis of logic, evidence, propaganda devices, and language	☐	☐	☐	☐	☐
Explains and advances opinions by citing evidence and referring to sources	☐	☐	☐	☐	☐
Summarizes the main points of a discussion, orally and in writing, specifying areas of agreement and disagreement and paraphrasing contributions	☐	☐	☐	☐	☐
Displays and maintains facial expressions, body language, and other response cues that indicate respect for the speaker and attention to the discussion	☐	☐	☐	☐	☐
Participates in a discussion without dominating	☐	☐	☐	☐	☐
Distinguishes between supported and unsupported statements	☐	☐	☐	☐	☐
Describes the role of communication in everyday situations (e.g., advertising, informal social, business, formal social)	☐	☐	☐	☐	☐
Can use persuasion, argumentation, and debate as essential oral skills	☐	☐	☐	☐	☐
Applies assessment criteria to self-evaluation of oral presentations	☐	☐	☐	☐	☐
Constructs and presents a coherent argument, summarizing and then refuting opposing positions, and citing persuasive evidence	☐	☐	☐	☐	☐
Participates effectively in question-and-answer sessions following presentations	☐	☐	☐	☐	☐
Demonstrates the ability to debate an issue from either side	☐	☐	☐	☐	☐
Interprets literary works orally, citing textual data in support of assertions	☐	☐	☐	☐	☐
Synthesizes and presents results of research projects, accurately summarizing and illustrating the main ideas, using appropriate technological aids, and offering support for the conclusions	☐	☐	☐	☐	☐
Speaks fluently with varied inflection and effective eye contact, enunciating clearly at an appropriate rate and volume	☐	☐	☐	☐	☐

Ninth to Twelfth Grade Oral Language Skills *(continued)*

	0	1	2	3	4
Distinguishes between literal and connotative meanings	☐	☐	☐	☐	☐
Distinguishes between relevant and irrelevant information	☐	☐	☐	☐	☐
Detects and evaluates a speaker's bias	☐	☐	☐	☐	☐
Is aware of and tries to control counterproductive emotional responses to a speaker or ideas conveyed in a discussion	☐	☐	☐	☐	☐
Performs various roles in a discussion including leader, participant, and moderator	☐	☐	☐	☐	☐
Demonstrates the ability to extend a discussion by adding relevant information or asking pertinent questions	☐	☐	☐	☐	☐
Conveys criticism in a respectful and supportive way	☐	☐	☐	☐	☐

INDEX